Basic Radiographic
Positioning and Anatomy

BASIC RADIOGRAPHIC

POSITIONING

AND ANATOMY

G. A. Bell BSC, TDCR, Cert.Ed, SRR
Principal, Schools of Radiography
The Leicester Royal Infirmary

and

D. B. L. Finlay MRCP, FRCR
Consultant Radiologist
The Leicester Royal Infirmary
and Honorary Lecturer
University of Leicester

Baillière Tindall
London · Philadelphia · Toronto · Sydney · Tokyo

Baillière Tindall   24–28 Oval Road
W. B. Saunders   London NW1 7DX

The Curtis Center
Independence Square West
Philadelphia, PA 19106–3399, USA

55 Horner Avenue
Toronto, Ontario M8Z 4X6, Canada

Harcourt Brace Jovanovich Group (Australia) Pty Ltd
30–52 Smidmore Steet
Marrickville
NSW 2204, Australia

Harcourt Brace Jovanovich Japan Inc.
Ichibancho Central Building, 22–1 Ichibancho
Chiyoda-ku, Tokyo 102, Japan

First published 1986
Third Printing 1993

Typeset by Photo-Graphics, Honiton, Devon.
Printed and bound in Great Britain
by The Alden Press, Oxford.

British Library Cataloguing in Publication Data

Bell, G. A.
    Basic radiographic positioning and anatomy.
    1. Diagnosis, Radioscopic
    I. Title   II. Finlay, D.B.L.
    616.07'57   RC78

    ISBN 0–7020–0978–4

CONTENTS

ACKNOWLEDGEMENTS

Our thanks are due to Mr Graham Tuppen at the Leicester Royal Infirmary for assistance with positioning, to Mrs Mary Baker and Mr Colin Best at the Northampton General Hospital, Mr Geoff Glover at the Leicester General Hospital and Mrs Carol Oley at the Derbyshire Royal Infirmary for reading the draft manuscript and offering much helpful advice, and to Mrs Lynn Towers for typing the manuscript.

The basic design and layout of the book were devised by Mr Russell Kightley at the Leicester Royal Infirmary.

This book is intended to be a useful practical guide for the student radiographer, and combines basic radiographic techniques and radiographic anatomical appearances in a simple, easy-to-use form. Each of the 126 routine positions included from the skeletal system, thorax and abdomen is dealt with by region in a systematic way using the same format throughout. The patient positions and associated radiographic anatomy are illustrated by line diagrams, and each technique is described in a concise manner so as to be easily understood with the essential facts readily available. The placing of an anatomical marker, the collimation of the x-ray beam and the application of radiation protection to the patient are all emphasized. For most projections details are included of exposure conditions, additional or modified techniques and other information relevant to the examination. Space is provided for readers to add their own notes and exposure factors to accompany each projection described. A chart containing typical exposure factors is included in an Appendix, although this should only be regarded as a guide. Although non-screen film is suggested as an alternative for a number of projections mainly for the upper and lower limbs it should be noted that this type of film may not be available in many X-ray departments.

The following abbreviations and terms are used throughout the book. (Additional abbreviations, which are used only in the Appendix, are explained in the footnotes to the Appendix.)

kVp, tube kilovoltage peak

mAs, tube milliampere seconds

fss, focal spot size

ffd, focus–film distance

Film/screen, film/screen combination

Grid, stationary grid or bucky

SECTION 1

UPPER LIMB

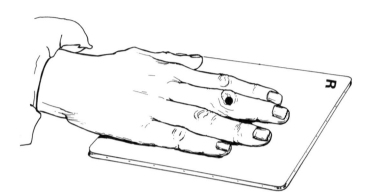

Dorsipalmar (posteroanterior) view of right fingers

Equipment required   13 × 18 cm detail screens cassette or non-screen film.
Lead rubber backing sheet for non-screen film.
Sandbag.
Lead protective waist apron.

Patient position   Seat the patient alongside the x-ray couch. Place palmar aspect of fingers under examination on film. Separate fingers slightly. Include either the thumb or little finger. Immobilize hand and wrist. Place anatomical marker, collimate beam and apply protection.

Centring point   At the level of the proximal interphalangeal joint of the finger or fingers under examination.

Direction of central ray   Vertical at 90° to the film.

Special note   The centring point for the middle finger is shown.

R

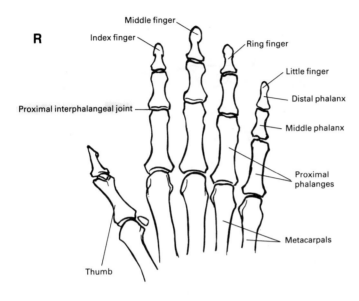

Middle finger
Index finger
Ring finger
Little finger
Distal phalanx
Proximal interphalangeal joint
Middle phalanx
Proximal phalanges
Metacarpals
Thumb

Notes

kVp
mAs
fss
ffd
Film/screen
Grid

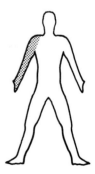

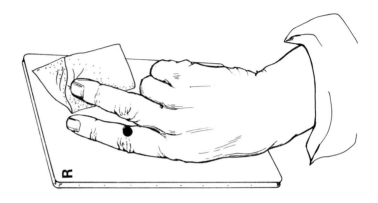

Lateral view of right index and middle fingers

Equipment required   13 × 18 cm detail screens cassette or
non-screen film.
Lead rubber backing sheet for
non-screen film.
Sandbag.
Small foam pad.
Lead protective waist apron.

Patient position   Seat the patient alongside the x-ray couch.
Rotate the hand medially and place lateral border of index
finger on film. Extend and separate index and middle fingers.
Support middle finger with foam pad. Flex other fingers.
Immobilize the hand and wrist. Place anatomical marker,
collimate beam and apply protection.

Centring point   Proximal interphalangeal joint of the finger
under examination.

Direction of central ray   Vertical at 90° to the film.

Special note   The centring point for the index finger is
shown.

R

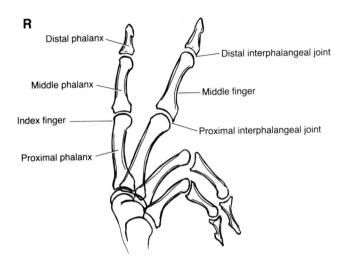

Distal phalanx

Distal interphalangeal joint

Middle phalanx

Middle finger

Index finger

Proximal interphalangeal joint

Proximal phalanx

Notes

kVp
mAs
fss
ffd
Film/screen
Grid

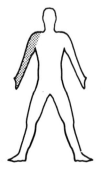

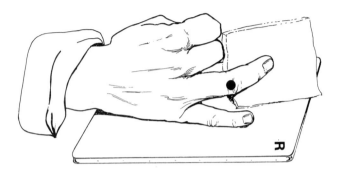

Lateral view of right ring and little fingers

Equipment required 13 × 18 cm detail screens cassette or non-screen film.
Lead rubber backing sheet for non-screen film.
Sandbag.
Small foam pad.
Lead protective apron.

Patient position Seat the patient alongside the x-ray couch. Place medial border of hand on film. Extend and separate ring and little fingers. Support ring finger with foam pad. Flex other fingers. Immobilize the hand and wrist. Place anatomical marker, collimate beam and apply protection.

Centring point Proximal interphalangeal joint of the finger under examination.

Direction of centring ray Vertical at 90° to the film.

Special note The centring point for the ring finger is shown.

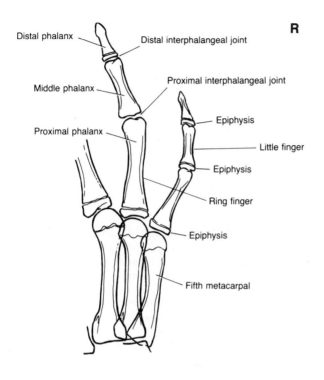

R

Distal phalanx

Distal interphalangeal joint

Middle phalanx

Proximal interphalangeal joint

Proximal phalanx

Epiphysis

Little finger

Epiphysis

Ring finger

Epiphysis

Fifth metacarpal

Notes

kVp
mAs
fss
ffd
Film/screen
Grid

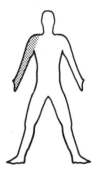

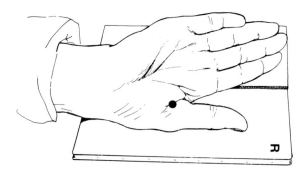

Anteroposterior view of right thumb

Equipment required   13 × 18 cm detail screens cassette or non-screen film split with sheet of lead rubber.
Lead rubber backing sheet for non-screen film.
Sandbag.
Lead protective waist apron.

Patient position   Seat the patient alongside the x-ray couch with shoulder at couch level. Extend hand, wrist and forearm. Rotate arm medially until posterior aspect of thumb is resting on the film. Ensure that the hypothenar eminence is not superimposed over the first metacarpal. Immobilize hand and wrist. Place anatomical marker, collimate beam and apply protection.

Centring point   Metacarpophalangeal joint of thumb.

Direction of central ray   Vertical at 90° to the film.

Special features   Include the whole of the first metacarpal for possible fracture at the base (Bennett's fracture).

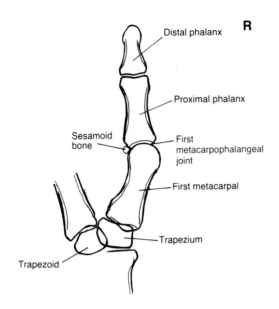

R

Distal phalanx

Proximal phalanx

Sesamoid bone

First metacarpophalangeal joint

First metacarpal

Trapezium

Trapezoid

Notes

kVp
mAs
fss
ffd
Film/screen
Grid

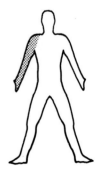

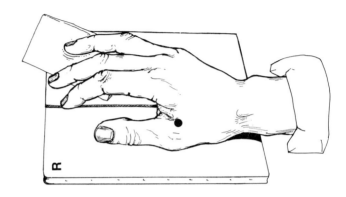

Lateral view of right thumb

Equipment required   13 × 18 cm detail screens cassette or non-screen film split with sheet of lead rubber.
Lead rubber backing sheet for non-screen film.
Foam pad.
Sandbag.
Lead protective waist apron.

Patient position   Seat the patient alongside the x-ray couch. Extend hand and wrist. Place palmar aspect of hand on film and separate thumb. Raise palm on pad until thumb is in true lateral position. Immobilize hand and wrist. Place anatomical marker, collimate beam and apply protection.

Centring point   Metacarpophalangeal joint of thumb.

Direction of central ray   Vertical at 90° to the film.

Special features   Include the whole of the first metacarpal for possible fracture at the base (Bennett's fracture).

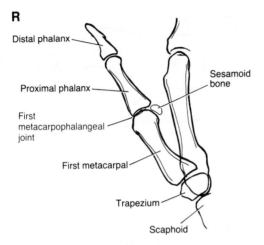

R

Distal phalanx

Proximal phalanx

First
metacarpophalangeal
joint

First metacarpal

Trapezium

Scaphoid

Sesamoid
bone

Notes

kVp
mAs
fss
ffd
Film/screen
Grid

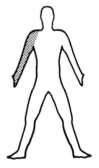

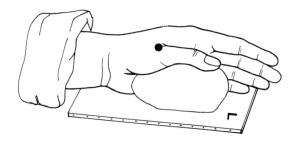

Posteroanterior view of left thumb

Equipment required 13 × 18 cm detail screens cassette or non-screen film.
Lead rubber backing sheet for non-screen film.
Sandbag.
Small foam pad.
Radiopaque marker.
Lead protective waist apron.

Patient position Seat the patient alongside the x-ray couch. Extend hand, wrist and forearm. Place medial border of hand on film and rotate hand medially until palmar aspect is at 15° to film. Extend thumb and rest on a small radiolucent pad. Avoid exerting any pressure on the thenar eminence. Immobilize, place anatomical marker, collimate beam and apply protection.

Centring point Metacarpophalangeal joint of thumb.

Direction of central ray Vertical at 90° to the film.

Special note Place radiopaque marker over site of entry of foreign body and leave in place for casualty officer. Increase the focus–film distance to 120 cm to compensate for the large object–film distance. This projection may also be used instead of the anteroposterior for serious injury.

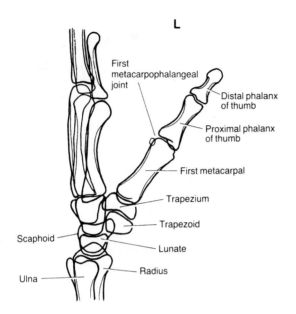

L

First metacarpophalangeal joint

Distal phalanx of thumb

Proximal phalanx of thumb

First metacarpal

Trapezium

Trapezoid

Scaphoid

Lunate

Ulna

Radius

Notes

kVp
mAs
fss
ffd
Film/screen
Grid

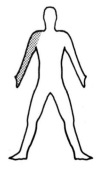

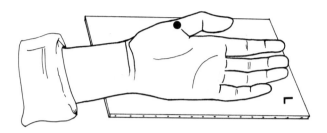

Mediolateral view of left thumb

Equipment required   13 × 18 cm detail screens cassette or non-screen film.
Lead rubber backing sheet for non-screen film.
Sandbag.
Radiopaque marker.
Lead protective waist apron.

Patient position   Seat the patient alongside the x-ray couch. Extend hand, wrist and forearm. Place the medial border of the hand on the film and rotate the hand laterally until the palm is at 45°. Avoid exerting any pressure on the thenar eminence. Immobilize, place anatomical marker, collimate beam and apply protection.

Centring point   Metacarpophalangeal joint of the thumb.

Direction of central ray   Vertical at 90° to the film.

Special note   Place radiopaque marker over site of entry of foreign body and leave in place for casualty officer. Increase the focus–film distance to 120 cm to compensate for the large object–film distance. This projection may also be used instead of the lateral for serious injury to the palmar aspect of the thumb.

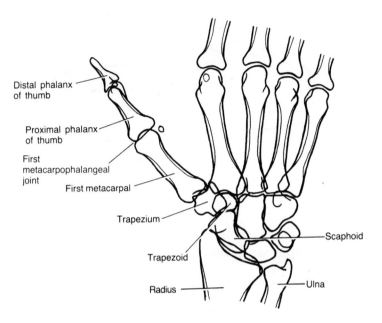

Distal phalanx
of thumb

Proximal phalanx
of thumb

First
metacarpophalangeal
joint

First metacarpal

Trapezium

Trapezoid

Radius

Scaphoid

Ulna

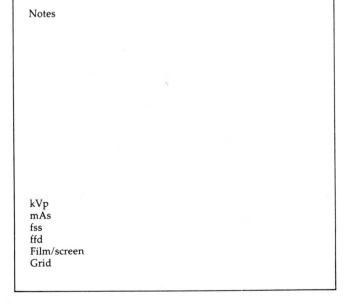

Notes

kVp
mAs
fss
ffd
Film/screen
Grid

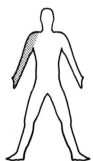

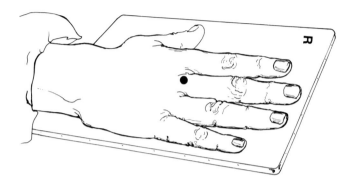

Dorsipalmar (posteroanterior) view of right hand

Equipment required   18 × 24 cm detail screens cassette or non-screen film.
(24 × 30 cm if split and sheet of lead rubber.)
Lead rubber backing sheet for non-screen film.
Sandbag.
Lead protective waist apron.

Patient position   Seat the patient alongside the x-ray couch. Extend hand, wrist and forearm in a straight line. Place palmar aspect of hand on film to include the wrist joint. Extend fingers, separate slightly and space evenly. Immobilize lower forearm. Place anatomical marker, collimate beam and apply protection.

Centring point   Head of third metacarpal.

Direction of central ray   Vertical at 90° to the film.

Special features   If the patient is unable to extend the fingers fully, or in the event of serious injury, the hand may need to be examined anteroposterior. To demonstrate bone age a dorsipalmar view of the left hand is usually taken.

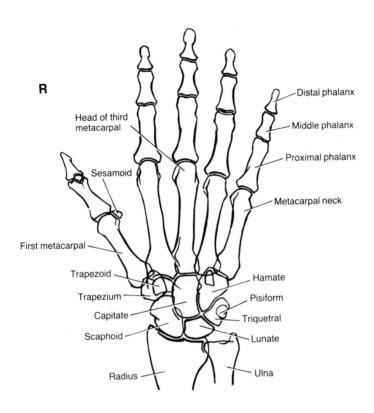

R

Distal phalanx

Head of third metacarpal

Middle phalanx

Sesamoid

Proximal phalanx

Metacarpal neck

First metacarpal

Trapezoid

Hamate

Trapezium

Pisiform

Capitate

Triquetral

Scaphoid

Lunate

Radius

Ulna

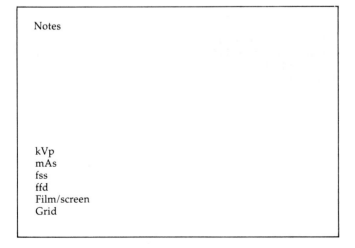

Notes

kVp
mAs
fss
ffd
Film/screen
Grid

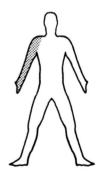

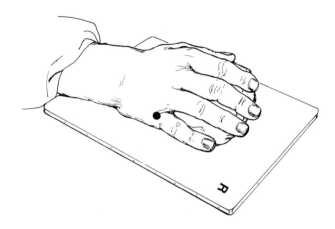

Dorsipalmar oblique view of right hand

Equipment required   18 × 24 cm detail screens cassette or non-screen film.
(24 × 30 cm if split and sheet of lead rubber.)
Lead rubber backing sheet for non-screen film.
Small foam pad.
Sandbag.
Lead protective waist apron.

Patient position   Seat the patient alongside the x-ray couch. Extend hand, wrist and forearm in a straight line. Place palm of hand on film to include the wrist joint. Raise thumb until palm is at 45° to film. Separate and slightly flex fingers and thumb and support on pad. Immobilize forearm. Place anatomical marker, collimate beam and apply protection.

Centring point   Head of the fifth metatarsal.

Direction of central ray   Vertical at 90° to film.

Special features

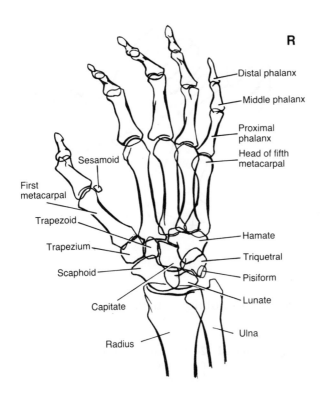

R

Distal phalanx

Middle phalanx

Proximal phalanx

Head of fifth metacarpal

Sesamoid

First metacarpal

Trapezoid

Trapezium

Scaphoid

Capitate

Radius

Hamate

Triquetral

Pisiform

Lunate

Ulna

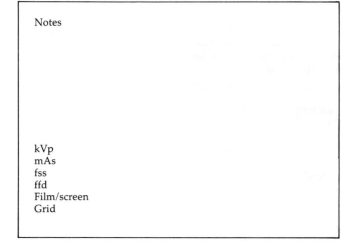

Notes

kVp
mAs
fss
ffd
Film/screen
Grid

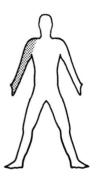

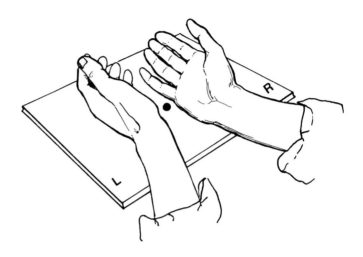

Anteroposterior oblique (ballcatcher) view of both hands

Equipment required   24 × 30 cm detail screens cassette or non-screen film.
Lead rubber backing sheet for non-screen film.
Sandbags.
Lead protective waist apron.

Patient position   Seat the patient at one end of the x-ray couch. Cup the hand as if catching a ball and rest the mediodorsal aspect of each hand on the film side by side. Immobilize hands and wrists. Place anatomical marker, collimate beam and apply protection.

Centring point   Midway between the hands at the level of the heads of the fifth metacarpals.

Direction of central ray   Vertical at 90° to the film.

Special features   This projection will demonstrate the metacarpophalangeal joint spaces for pathological changes such as rheumatoid arthritis. A bone phantom may be included on the film to assist in the assessment of bone density.

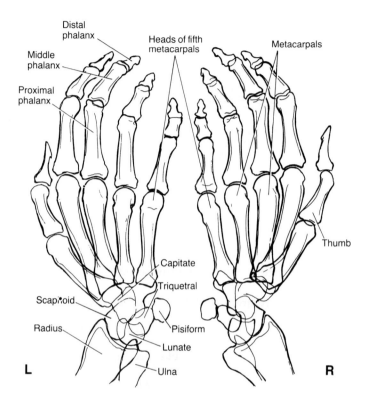

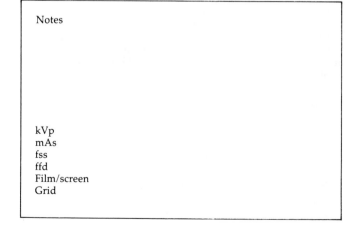

Notes

kVp
mAs
fss
ffd
Film/screen
Grid

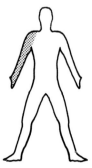

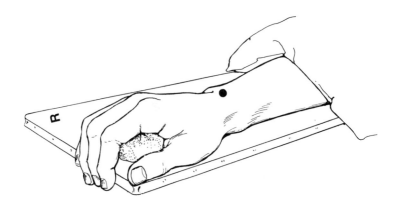

Posteroanterior view of right wrist

Equipment required   18 × 24 cm detail screens cassette or
non-screen film.
(24 × 30 cm film if split with sheet of
lead rubber.)
Lead rubber backing sheet for
non-screen film.
Small foam pad.
Sandbag.
Lead protective waist apron.

Patient position   Seat the patient alongside the x-ray couch.
Rest palm, wrist and lower forearm in a straight line on film.
Place small pad under metacarpophalangeal joints of hand to
maintain wrist in close contact with film. Immobilize the wrist
and forearm. Place anatomical marker, collimate beam and
apply protection.

Centring point   Midway between the ulnar and radial styloid
processes.

Direction of central ray   Vertical at 90° to the film.

Special features   If the wrist is in plaster of Paris cast, use
detail or fast screens cassette with an appropriate alteration in
exposure factors.

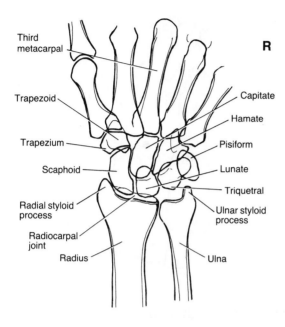

R

Third metacarpal

Trapezoid

Trapezium

Scaphoid

Radial styloid process

Radiocarpal joint

Radius

Capitate

Hamate

Pisiform

Lunate

Triquetral

Ulnar styloid process

Ulna

Notes

kVp
mAs
fss
ffd
Film/screen
Grid

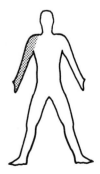

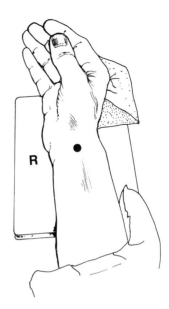

Lateral view of right wrist

Equipment required   18 × 24 cm detail screens cassette or
non-screen film.
(24 × 30 cm film if split.)
Lead rubber backing sheet for
non-screen film.
Foam pad.
Sandbag.
Lead protective waist apron.

Patient position   Seat the patient alongside the x-ray couch.
Extend hand, wrist and forearm. Rotate the forearm into the
lateral position and rest the fifth finger and medial aspect of
hand and lower forearm in a straight line on film. Ensure
ulnar and radial styloid processes are vertically superimposed
by 5° posterior rotation of hand. Support back of hand with
pad and immobilize forearm. Place anatomical marker,
collimate beam and apply protection.

Centring point   Radial styloid process.

Direction of central ray   Vertical at 90° to film.

Special features   If the wrist is in a plaster of Paris cast, use
detail or fast screens cassette with an appropriate alteration in
exposure factors.

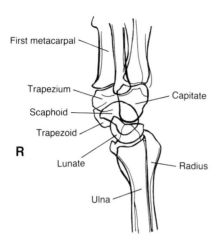

First metacarpal

Trapezium

Scaphoid

Trapezoid

R

Lunate

Ulna

Capitate

Radius

Notes

kVp
mAs
fss
ffd
Film/screen
Grid

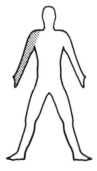

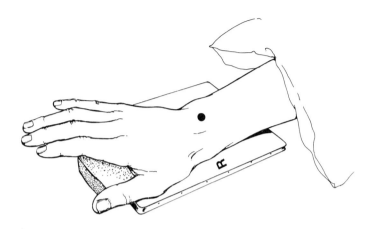

Posteroanterior view of right wrist with ulnar deviation

Equipment required   18 × 24 cm detail screens cassette or non-screen film.
(24 × 30 cm if split and sheet of lead rubber.)
Lead rubber backing sheet for non-screen film.
Small foam pad.
Sandbag.
Lead protective waist apron.

Patient position   Seat the patient alongside the x-ray couch. Rest palm, wrist and lower forearm on film with ulnar deviation of hand. Place small pad under metacarpophalangeal joints of hand to maintain wrist in close contact with film. Immobilize forearm. Place anatomical marker, collimate beam and apply protection.

Centring point   Midway between ulnar and radial styloid processes.

Direction of central ray   Vertical at 90° to the film.

Special features   It is important that the patient should be allowed to ulnar deviate the wrist without the use of any force. It may be necessary to examine the patient again at least 14 days after the initial examination in order to demonstrate a fractured scaphoid radiographically.

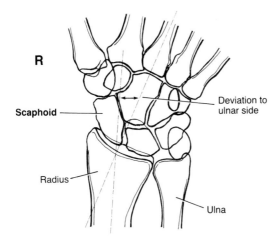

R

Scaphoid

Deviation to
ulnar side

Radius

Ulna

Notes

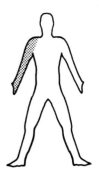

kVp
mAs
fss
ffd
Film/screen
Grid

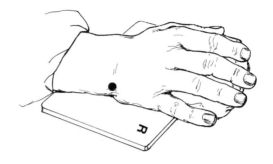

Oblique view of right wrist for scaphoid

Equipment required   18 × 24 cm detail screens cassette or
non-screen film.
Lead rubber backing sheet for
non-screen film.
Small foam pad.
Sandbag.
Lead protective waist apron.

Patient position   Seat the patient alongside the x-ray couch.
From the posteroanterior position rotate the hand laterally
until the palmar aspect is at 45° to the film. Place a small
radiolucent pad under the thumb and fingers. Immobilize
forearm. Place anatomical marker, collimate beam and apply
protection.

Centring point   Ulnar styloid process.

Direction of central ray   Vertical at 90° to the film.

Special features   It may be necessary to examine the patient
again at least 14 days after the initial examination in order to
demonstrate a fractured scaphoid radiographically.

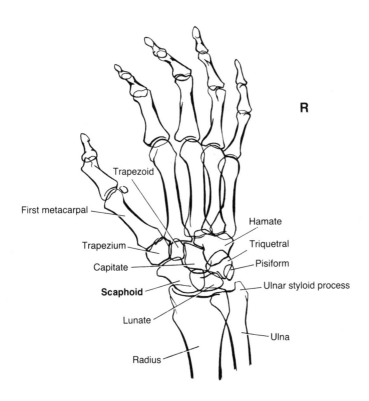

R

First metacarpal

Trapezoid

Trapezium

Capitate

Scaphoid

Lunate

Radius

Hamate

Triquetral

Pisiform

Ulnar styloid process

Ulna

Notes

kVp
mAs
fss
ffd
Film/screen
Grid

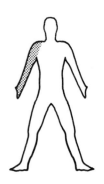

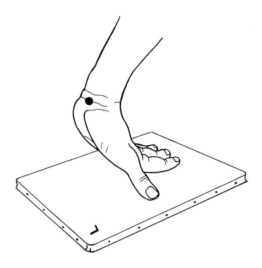

Superoinferior (axial) view of left wrist for carpal tunnel

Equipment required   18 × 24 cm detail screens cassette or non-screen film.
Lead rubber backing sheet for non-screen film.
Foam pad.
Lead protective waist apron.

Patient position   Stand the patient with the back to the x-ray couch and arm extended. Flex the elbow and wrist, and with the fingers and thumb well separated press the hand palm down on to a film near the edge of the couch. Ensure that the carpal region is in profile. Immobilize the hand with a foam pad if necessary. Place anatomical marker, collimate beam and apply protection.

Centring point   Midcarpal region.

Direction of central ray   Vertical at 90° to film.

Special note   The patient should wear the lead protective waist apron at the back.

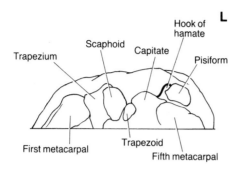

L

Trapezium   Scaphoid   Capitate   Hook of hamate   Pisiform

First metacarpal   Trapezoid   Fifth metacarpal

Notes

kVp
mAs
fss
ffd
Film/screen
Grid

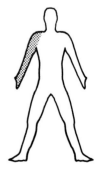

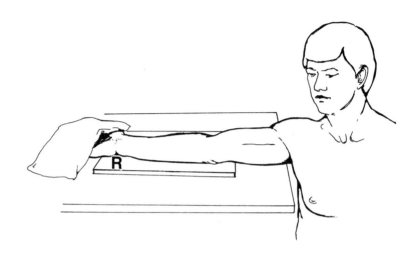

Anteroposterior view of right forearm

Equipment required   18 × 40 cm detail screens cassette or non-screen film.
(30 × 40 cm if split with sheet of lead rubber.)
Lead rubber backing sheet for non-screen film.
Sandbag.
Lead protective waist apron.

Patient position   Seat the patient alongside the x-ray couch with shoulder at couch level. Place forearm fully supinated with elbow extended. Include wrist and elbow if possible. Immobilize hand with sandbag. Place anatomical marker, collimate beam and apply protection.

Centring point   Anterior aspect of the middle of the forearm, midway between the wrist and elbow.

Direction of central ray   Vertical at 90° to film.

Special features

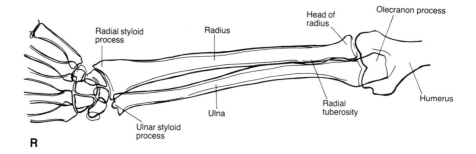

R

Notes

kVp
mAs
fss
ffd
Film/screen
Grid

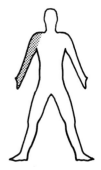

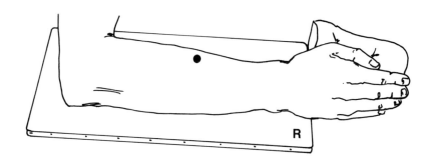

Lateral view of right forearm

Equipment required   18 × 40 cm detail screens cassette or non-screen film.
(30 × 40 cm if split and sheet of lead rubber.)
Lead rubber backing sheet for non-screen film.
Sandbag.
Lead protective waist apron.

Patient position   Seat the patient alongside the x-ray couch. Lower shoulder of affected side to same level as forearm. Flex elbow at 90°. Place medial border of forearm on film. Include wrist and elbow if possible. Immobilize hand with sandbag. Place anatomical marker, collimate beam and apply protection.

Centring point   Lateral aspect of the forearm over the radius midway between the wrist and elbow.

Direction of central ray   Vertical at 90° to film.

Special features

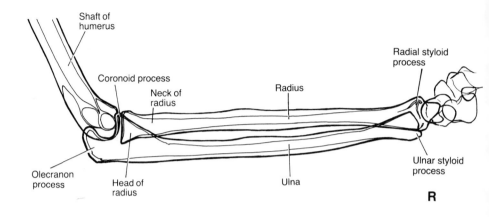

Shaft of humerus

Coronoid process

Neck of radius

Radius

Radial styloid process

Olecranon process

Head of radius

Ulna

Ulnar styloid process

R

Notes

kVp
mAs
fss
ffd
Film/screen
Grid

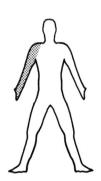

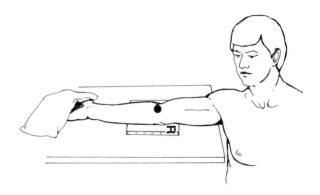

Anteroposterior view of right elbow

Equipment required 18 × 24 cm detail screens cassette or non-screen film.
(24 × 30 cm film if split and sheet of lead rubber.)
Lead rubber backing sheet for non-screen film.
Sandbag.
Lead protective waist apron.

Patient position Seat the patient sideways alongside the x-ray couch, with the shoulder at couch level. Fully supinate forearm, extend elbow and rest on film. Ensure that the patient's thumb is touching the couch top if possible. Place anatomical marker, collimate beam and apply protection.

Centring point In the midline 2.5 cm distal to a line joining the epicondyles of the humerus.

Direction of central ray Vertical at 90° to film.

Special features It is important after injury not to extend the elbow if this causes pain, because of the possible presence of a supracondylar fracture. A detail screens cassette should be used if the exposure with non-screen film is unduly long.

Modified anteroposterior If the patient cannot fully extend the elbow due to injury, then rest the olecranon on the film with the forearm and humerus both supported at an angle of 45° to the film. Centre to the midline of the crease of the elbow.

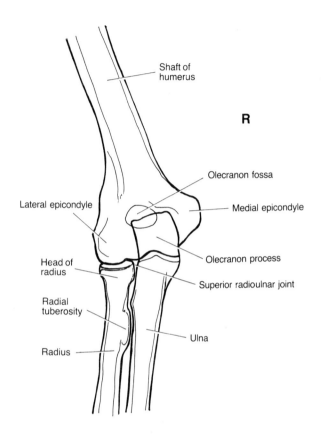

Shaft of
humerus

R

Olecranon fossa

Lateral epicondyle

Medial epicondyle

Olecranon process

Head of
radius

Superior radioulnar joint

Radial
tuberosity

Ulna

Radius

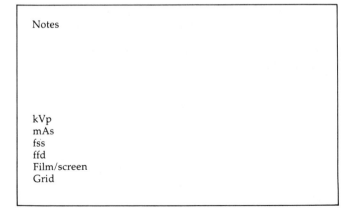

Notes

kVp
mAs
fss
ffd
Film/screen
Grid

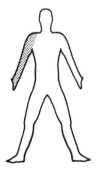

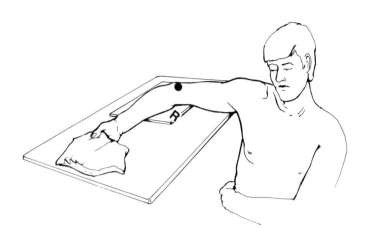

Lateral view of right elbow

Equipment required   18 × 24 cm detail screens cassette or non-screen film.
(24 × 30 cm film if split and sheet of lead rubber.)
Lead rubber backing sheet for non-screen film.
Sandbag.
Lead protective waist apron.

Patient position   Seat the patient sideways alongside the x-ray couch with shoulder, elbow and hand at the same level. Flex elbow 90° and rotate forearm into true lateral position with thumb uppermost. Rest medial border of elbow on film. Immobilize hand and wrist. Place anatomical marker, collimate beam and apply protection.

Centring point   Lateral epicondyle of humerus.

Direction of central ray   Vertical at 90° to film.

Special features   After injury the lateral should be taken first as it usually causes less pain, and further views taken accordingly. A detail screens cassette should be used if the exposure with non-screen film would be unduly long.

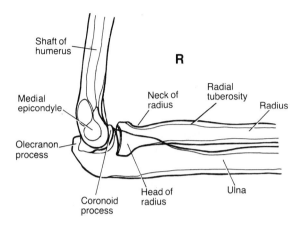

Shaft of humerus

R

Medial epicondyle

Neck of radius

Radial tuberosity

Radius

Olecranon process

Coronoid process

Head of radius

Ulna

Notes

kVp
mAs
fss
ffd
Film/screen
Grid

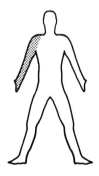

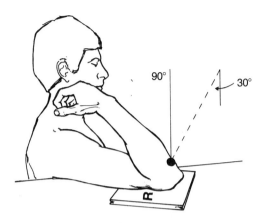

Axial view of right elbow

Equipment required   18 × 24 cm detail screens cassette or
non-screen film.
Lead rubber backing sheet for
non-screen film.
Lead protective waist apron.

Patient position   Seat the patient alongside the x-ray couch
with shoulder at couch level. Flex the elbow so that the hand
is in contact with the shoulder. Rest the elbow on the film
with the upper arm at couch level. Place anatomical marker,
collimate beam and apply protection.

Centring point   In the midline 5 cm distal to the olecranon
process.

Direction of central ray   Vertical at 90° to film to demonstrate
the olecranon process.

Special features   The central ray may be angled 30° towards
the shoulder to demonstrate the radiohumeral joint space.
This projection is also of value for a suspected supracondylar
fracture when removal of the arm from sling is not advisable.

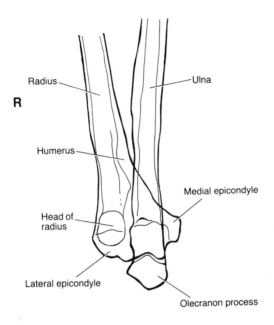

R

Radius

Ulna

Humerus

Medial epicondyle

Head of radius

Lateral epicondyle

Olecranon process

Notes

kVp
mAs
fss
ffd
Film/screen
Grid

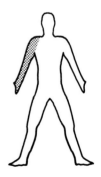

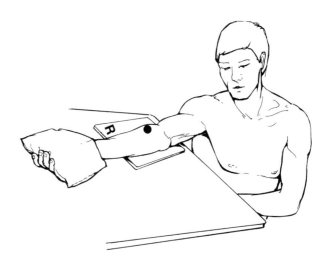

Oblique view of right elbow

Equipment required   18 × 24 cm detail screens cassette or
non-screen film.
Lead rubber backing sheet for
non-screen film.
Sandbag.
Lead protective waist apron.

Patient position   Seat the patient sideways alongside the
x-ray couch with the shoulder at couch level. Extend elbow
with forearm fully supinated. Rotate the arm outward slightly,
to separate the head of radius and ulna, and rest on film.
Immobilize hand and wrist. Place anatomical marker,
collimate beam and apply protection.

Centring point   Head of radius.

Direction of central ray   Vertical at 90° to film.

Special features

Modified anteroposterior   This projection is also of value and
may be used instead of the oblique if preferred. Flex the
elbow at 90° and rest the olecranon on the film with the
forearm and humerus both supported at an angle of 45° to the
film. Centre to the head of the radius.

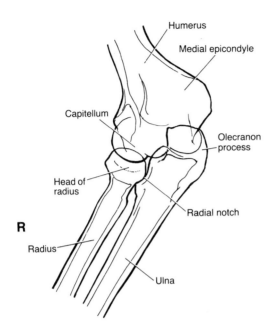

Humerus

Medial epicondyle

Capitellum

Olecranon process

Head of radius

Radial notch

R

Radius

Ulna

Notes

kVp
mAs
fss
ffd
Film/screen
Grid

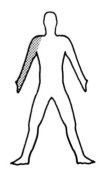

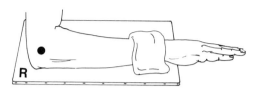

1. FOREARM PRONATED

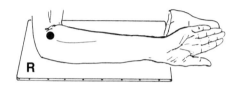

2. FOREARM MEDIALLY ROTATED

Lateral views of right elbow

Equipment required   24 × 30 cm detail screens cassette or non-screen film (split). Sheet of lead rubber. Lead rubber backing sheet for non-screen film. Sandbag. Lead protective waist apron.

Patient position   Seat the patient sideways alongside the x-ray couch with the shoulder, elbow and hand at couch level. Flex elbow at 90° and rest on film.

Lateral 1   Pronate forearm and rest the palm of the hand on the couch.
Lateral 2   Medially rotate the hand until the palm of the hand faces away from the trunk.

Immobilize forearm and wrist. Place anatomical markers, collimate beam and apply protection.

Centring point   Lateral epicondyle of the humerus.

Direction of central ray   Vertical at 90° to the film.

Special features   Both projections may be taken if required. These projections are an alternative to the oblique view of the elbow which may be the projection of choice for head of radius.

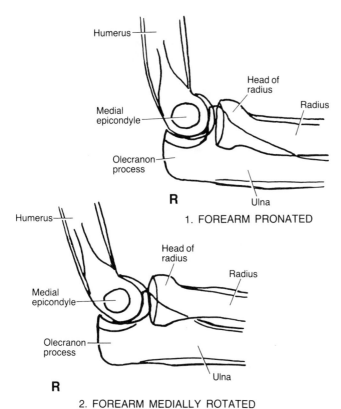

Humerus

Head of radius

Radius

Medial epicondyle

Olecranon process

R

Ulna

1. FOREARM PRONATED

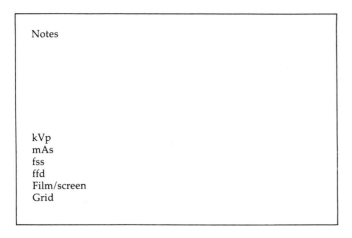

Humerus

Head of radius

Radius

Medial epicondyle

Olecranon process

R

Ulna

2. FOREARM MEDIALLY ROTATED

Notes

kVp
mAs
fss
ffd
Film/screen
Grid

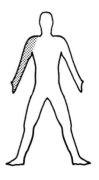

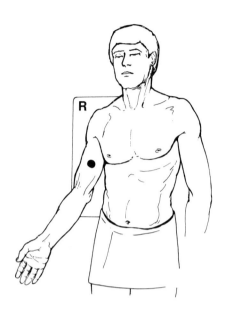

Anteroposterior view of right humerus

Equipment required   30 × 40 cm detail screens cassette.
Chest stand or upright cassette holder.
Lead protective waist apron.

Patient position   Stand or sit the patient facing towards the
x-ray tube. Rotate trunk slightly towards affected side. Place
the arm in the anatomical position. Rest the humerus against
the film to include shoulder and elbow. Place anatomical
marker, collimate beam and apply protection.

Centring point   Anterior aspect of humerus midway
between shoulder and elbow.

Direction of central ray   Horizontal at 90° to film.

Special features   Expose on arrested respiration. If the
patient is unable to stand or sit, or in the event of serious
injury, then the humerus should be examined with the
patient supine.

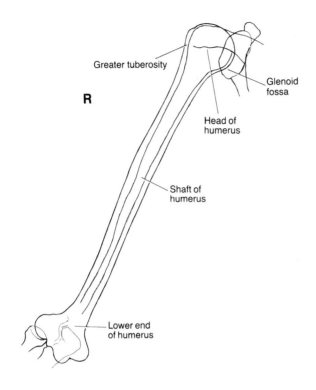

Greater tuberosity

R

Glenoid
fossa

Head of
humerus

Shaft of
humerus

Lower end
of humerus

Notes

kVp
mAs
fss
ffd
Film/screen
Grid

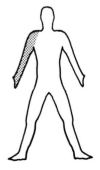

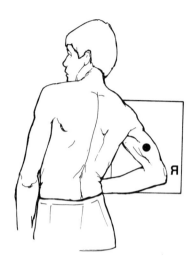

Lateral view of right humerus

Equipment required   30 × 40 cm detail screens cassette.
Chest stand or upright cassette holder.
Lead protective waist apron.

Patient position   Stand or sit the patient facing towards the
chest stand or upright cassette holder. Slightly abduct and
extend the arm and flex elbow. Rotate trunk away from
affected side until lateral aspect of the humerus rests on the
film. Include the shoulder and elbow. Place anatomical
marker, collimate beam and apply protection.

Centring point   Medial aspect of humerus midway between
shoulder and elbow.

Direction of central ray   Horizontal at 90° to film.

Special features   Expose on arrested respiration. If the
patient is unable to stand or sit, or in the event of serious
injury, the humerus should be examined with the patient
supine. Rotate trunk slightly to affected side. Flex elbow at 90°
and rest hand and forearm on the abdomen. Centre to lateral
aspect of humerus midway between shoulder and elbow with
the central ray vertical at 90° to film.

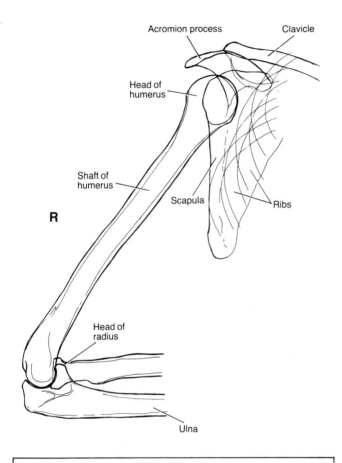

Acromion process

Clavicle

Head of
humerus

Shaft of
humerus

R

Scapula

Ribs

Head of
radius

Ulna

Notes

kVp
mAs
fss
ffd
Film/screen
Grid

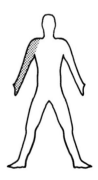

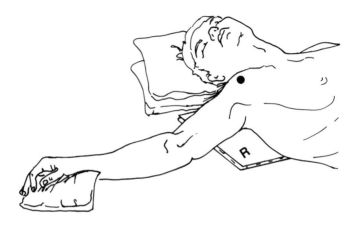

Anteroposterior view of right humerus for surgical neck

Equipment required 24 × 30 cm fast screens cassette.
Foam pads.
Sandbags.
Lead protective waist apron.

Patient position Keep patient supine on stretcher or trolley with head supported. Fully abduct arm if possible and support humerus in a comfortable position. Include shoulder and upper humerus. Immobilize the arm. Place anatomical marker, collimate beam and apply protection.

Centring point Head of humerus.

Direction of central ray Vertical at 90° to film.

Special features This examination will depend on the condition of the patient and should only be done if a medical officer is present.

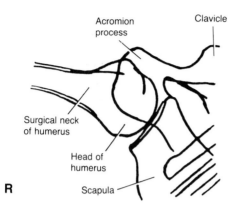

Acromion
process

Clavicle

Surgical neck
of humerus

Head of
humerus

R   Scapula

Notes

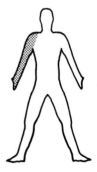

kVp
mAs
fss
ffd
Film/screen
Grid

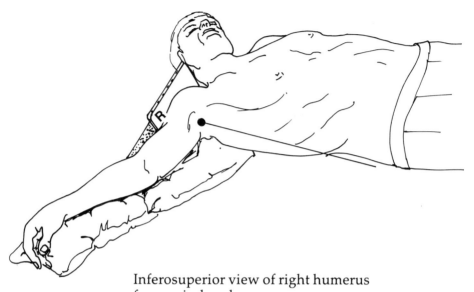

Inferosuperior view of right humerus
for surgical neck

Equipment required   24 × 30 cm fast screens cassette.
Foam pads.
Sandbags.
Lead protective waist apron.

Patient position   Keep the patient supine on stretcher or
trolley. Turn head away from affected side and support. Fully
abduct arm if possible, raise on pads and support in a
comfortable position. Vertically support cassette above
shoulder to include upper humerus. Immobilize the arm.
Place anatomical marker, collimate beam and apply
protection.

Centring point   Head of humerus through the axilla.

Direction of central ray   Horizontal and as close to the lateral
chest wall as possible.

Special features   This examination will depend on the
condition of the patient and should only be done if a medical
officer is present. It is preferable to take and view the
anteroposterior projection first. If a second projection is
required then the transthoracic lateral projection of the
shoulder may be a more suitable alternative.

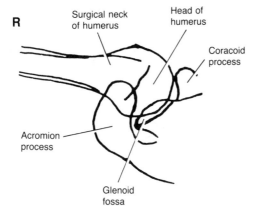

R

Surgical neck
of humerus

Head of
humerus

Coracoid
process

Acromion
process

Glenoid
fossa

Notes

kVp
mAs
fss
ffd
Film/screen
Grid

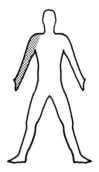

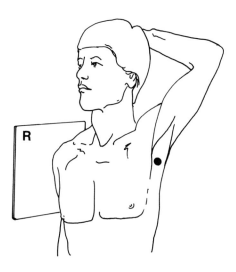

Transsthoracic lateral view of right shoulder for upper humerus

Equipment required   24 × 30 cm fast screens cassette (or gridded cassette).
Vertical bucky.
Lead protective waist apron.

Patient position   Stand or sit the patient in the true lateral position with the affected side towards the bucky top, and with the arm resting at the side of the body. Raise the arm on the unaffected side and rest over the patient's head. Immobilize the trunk. Place anatomical marker, collimate beam and apply protection.

Centring point   Head of humerus through the opposite axilla.

Direction of central ray   Horizontal at 90° to film.

Special features   Expose on arrested respiration. The tube kilovoltage should be at least 80 kVp. To diffuse the rib shadows (if the condition of the patient permits), expose during quiet respiration using a low mA setting and a long exposure time.

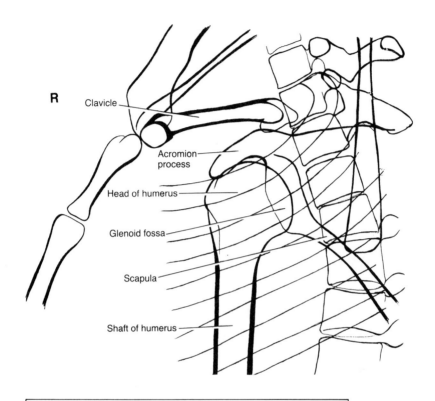

R

Clavicle

Acromion
process

Head of humerus

Glenoid fossa

Scapula

Shaft of humerus

Notes

kVp
mAs
fss
ffd
Film/screen
Grid

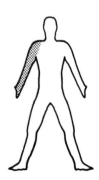

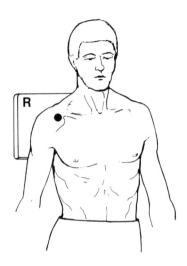

Anteroposterior view of right shoulder

Equipment required   24 × 30 cm detail screens cassette (or gridded cassette).
Chest stand or upright cassette holder (or vertical bucky).
Lead protective waist apron.

Patient position   Stand or lie the patient in the anteroposterior position. Rotate the trunk about 30° towards the affected side until the scapula is parallel to the film. Place the arm in the anatomical position and rest the shoulder on the cassette. Immobilize the shoulder. Place marker, collimate beam and apply protection.

Centring point   Anterior aspect of the shoulder over the coracoid process of the scapula.

Direction of central ray   Horizontal at 90° to film.

Special features   Expose during arrested respiration. If the patient is large then a secondary radiation grid should be used.

Modified anteroposterior   To demonstrate the glenohumeral joint space, rotate the trunk 25° towards the required shoulder. Partially abduct the arm with the elbow flexed. Centre to the head of the humerus.

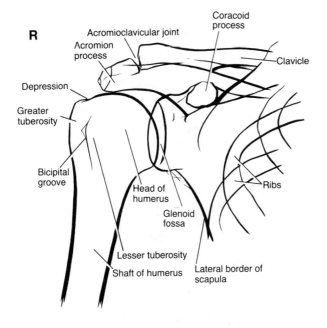

R

Coracoid process

Acromioclavicular joint

Acromion process

Clavicle

Depression

Greater tuberosity

Bicipital groove

Head of humerus

Glenoid fossa

Ribs

Lesser tuberosity

Shaft of humerus

Lateral border of scapula

Notes

kVp
mAs
fss
ffd
Film/screen
Grid

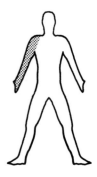

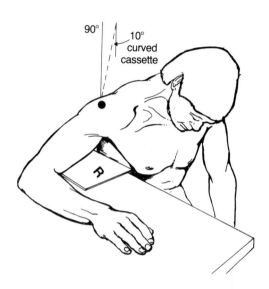

Axial (superoinferior) view of right shoulder

Equipment required   24 × 30 cm detail screens cassette or
curved cassette if available.
Lead rubber backing sheet.
Small localizing cone.
Lead protective waist apron.

Patient position   Seat the patient sideways alongside the
x-ray couch leaning slightly towards the couch. Abduct the
arm, flex the elbow at 90° and rest the forearm and hand on the
couch. Position the shoulder over the cassette to include the
glenohumeral joint. Place anatomical marker, collimate beam
using small localizing cone and apply protection.

Centring point   Head of humerus.

Direction of central ray   Vertical at 90° to film using a small
localizing cone.

Special features   Angle the tube 10° towards the head
(cephalad) to offset the angulation of the trunk if necessary.
Use fine focus and expose on arrested respiration. If a curved
cassette is available then lower the shoulder until the axilla is
in contact with the cassette. Centre to the acromion process
with the tube angled 10° towards the elbow.

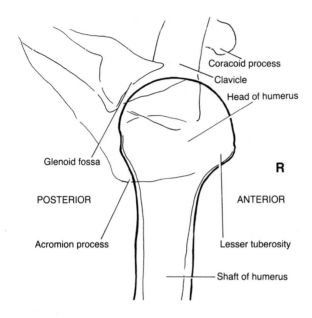

Coracoid process
Clavicle
Head of humerus

Glenoid fossa

R

POSTERIOR

ANTERIOR

Acromion process

Lesser tuberosity

Shaft of humerus

Notes

kVp
mAs
fss
ffd
Film/screen
Grid

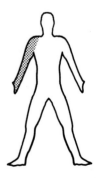

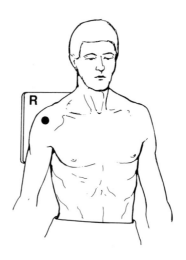

Anteroposterior view of right scapula

Equipment required   24 × 30 cm detail screens cassette.
Chest stand or upright cassette holder.
Lead protective waist apron.

Patient position   Stand or sit the patient facing towards the
x-ray tube. Rotate the trunk about 30° towards the affected
side until the scapula is parallel to the film. Place the arm in
the anatomical position and rest the scapula on the cassette.
Place anatomical marker, collimate beam and apply
protection.

Centring point   Head of humerus.

Direction of central ray   Horizontal at 90° to film.

Special features   Expose on arrested respiration.

R

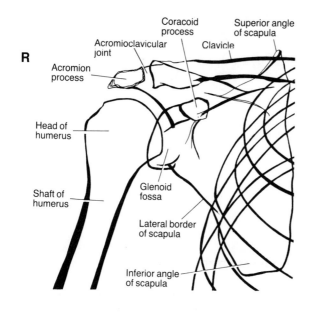

Coracoid process

Acromioclavicular joint

Acromion process

Clavicle

Superior angle of scapula

Head of humerus

Shaft of humerus

Glenoid fossa

Lateral border of scapula

Inferior angle of scapula

Notes

kVp
mAs
fss
ffd
Film/screen
Grid

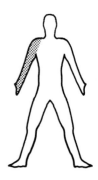

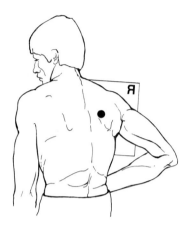

Lateral view of right scapula

Equipment required   24 × 30 cm detail or fast screens cassette (or gridded cassette). Chest stand or upright cassette holder (or vertical bucky). Lead protective waist apron.

Patient position   Stand or sit the patient facing towards the chest stand or upright cassette holder. Slightly abduct and extend humerus and flex elbow. Rotate the trunk until the blade of the scapula is at 90° to the film. Rest the shoulder on the cassette. Place anatomical marker, collimate beam and apply protection.

Centring point   Head of the humerus through the medial border of the scapula at the level of the fourth thoracic vertebra.

Direction of central ray   Horizontal at 90° to the film.

Special features   This projection may be used in preference to the transthoracic lateral projection of the shoulder to show dislocation of the head of the humerus. If the patient is large then a secondary radiation grid should be used.

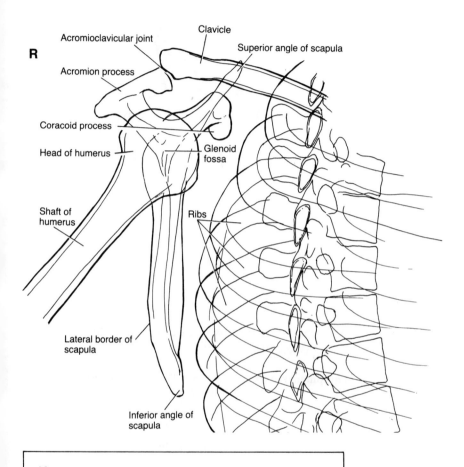

R

Acromioclavicular joint

Clavicle

Acromion process

Superior angle of scapula

Coracoid process

Head of humerus

Glenoid fossa

Shaft of humerus

Ribs

Lateral border of scapula

Inferior angle of scapula

Notes

kVp
mAs
fss
ffd
Film/screen
Grid

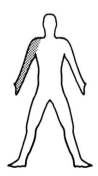

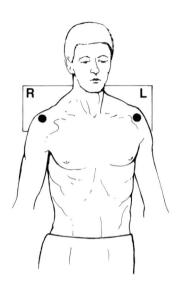

Anteroposterior view of both acromioclavicular joints (weight bearing)

Equipment required   Two 18 × 24 cm detail screens cassettes.
Two sandbags of equal weight.
Chest stand or upright cassette holder.
Lead protective waist apron.
Small localizing cone.

Patient position   Stand or sit the patient facing towards the x-ray tube with both arms in the anatomical position. Rest both shoulders against the cassettes held side by side in the upright cassette holder. Give the patient a sandbag to hold in each hand. Immobilize the patient. Place anatomical marker, collimate beam and apply protection.

Centring point   Each acromioclavicular joint in turn using a small localizing cone.

Direction of central ray   Horizontal at 90° to film.

Special note   Expose each side separately on arrested respiration.

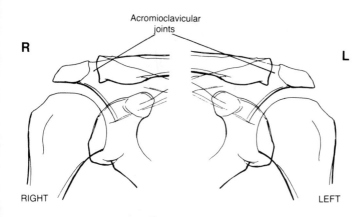

Acromioclavicular
joints

R

L

RIGHT

LEFT

Notes

kVp
mAs
fss
ffd
Film/screen
Grid

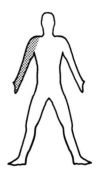

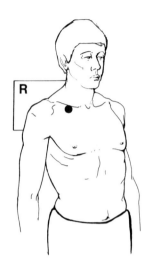

Anteroposterior view of right clavicle

Equipment required   24 × 30 cm detail screens cassette.
Chest stand or upright cassette holder.
Lead protective waist apron.

Patient position   Stand or sit the patient to face the x-ray
tube. Rest the shoulder of the affected side against the cassette
with the arm resting at the side of the body. Include the whole
of the clavicle. Place anatomical marker, collimate beam and
apply protection.

Centring point   Middle of the clavicle.

Direction of central ray   Horizontal at 90° to film.

Special features   Expose on arrested respiration. The
anteroposterior position is usually easier for an injured
patient than the posteroanterior.

Posteroanterior   If the condition of the patient permits, the
clavicle may be better demonstrated with this view. Stand or
sit the patient to face the cassette with the head turned away
from the affected side. Rotate the trunk slightly so that the
shoulder is in contact with the film. Rest the arm at the side of
the body. Centre to the superior angle of the scapula.

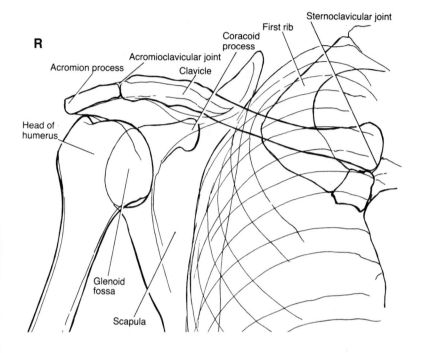

R

Sternoclavicular joint

First rib

Coracoid process

Acromioclavicular joint

Acromion process

Clavicle

Head of humerus

Glenoid fossa

Scapula

Notes

kVp
mAs
fss
ffd
Film/screen
Grid

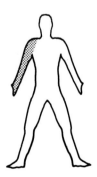

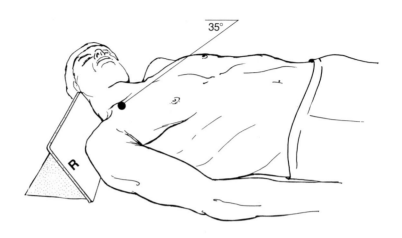

Inferosuperior view of right clavicle

Equipment required   24 × 30 cm detail screens cassette.
Large foam pad.
Lead protective waist apron.

Patient position   Lie the patient supine on the x-ray couch
with the arm on the affected side by the trunk with the palm
facing inwards. Turn head away from the affected side.
Support cassette at an angle in contact with posterior aspect of
shoulder using a large foam pad. Place anatomical marker,
collimate beam and apply protection.

Centring point   2.5 cm from sternal end of clavicle.

Direction of central ray   Angled at 35° to horizontal and 15°
laterally towards shoulder.

Special features   Expose on arrested respiration. If the
condition of the patient permits, the clavicle may also be
examined in the erect position using the chest stand with the
cassette holder angled forwards.

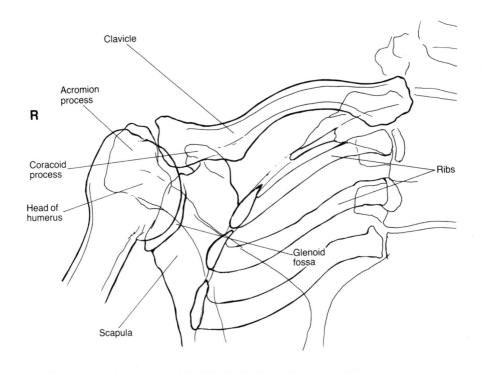

Clavicle

Acromion
process

R

Coracoid
process

Head of
humerus

Ribs

Glenoid
fossa

Scapula

Notes

kVp
mAs
fss
ffd
Film/screen
Grid

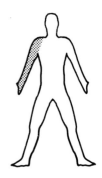

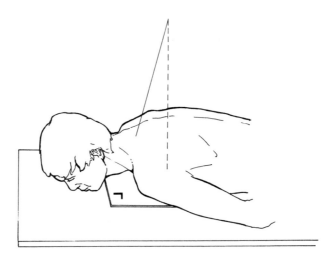

Posteroanterior view of both sternoclavicular joints

Equipment required   24 × 30 cm detail screens cassette.
Lead protective waist apron.
Small localizing cone.

Patient position   Lie the patient prone on the x-ray couch
with the sternoclavicular joints in contact with the centre of
the cassette. Place the arms by the side and the patient's chin
over the end of the cassette. Immobilize the patient. Place
anatomical marker, collimate beam and apply protection.

Centring point   To the suprasternal notch at the level of the
fourth thoracic vertebra.

Direction of central ray   Vertically over one shoulder and
then angled towards the midline using a small localizing cone.

Special features   Expose on arrested respiration. The patient
can be examined in the erect position, using the upright
cassette holder, if preferred.

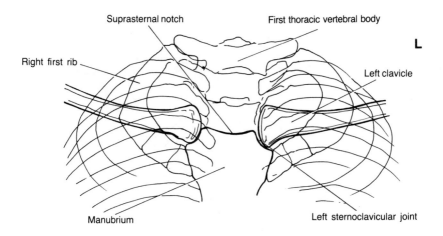

Suprasternal notch

First thoracic vertebral body

L

Right first rib

Left clavicle

Manubrium

Left sternoclavicular joint

(Note that the midline structures are slightly offset)

Notes

kVp
mAs
fss
ffd
Film/screen
Grid

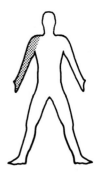

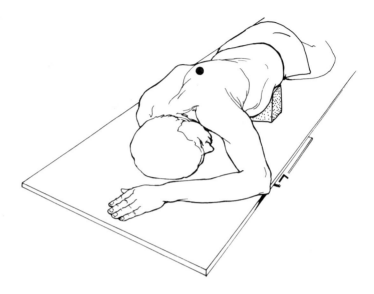

Right anterior oblique view of sternoclavicular joints

Equipment required   Two 24 × 30 cm detail screens cassette.
Table bucky.
Large foam pad.
Lead protective waist apron.

Patient position   Lie the patient prone on the x-ray couch
and rotate the trunk 45° to each side in turn and support. Place
the arm on the raised side above the head and the other by the
patient's side. Centre the sternoclavicular joint nearer the film
to the middle of the couch top and grid. Immobilize the
patient. Place anatomical marker, collimate beam and apply
protection.

Centring point   10 cm from the midline on the raised side at
the level of the fourth thoracic vertebra.

Direction of central ray   Vertical at 90° to film.

Special features   Expose each side separately on arrested
respiration. The patient can be examined in the erect position,
using the vertical bucky, if preferred. To diffuse the rib
shadows expose during quiet respiration using a low mA
setting and a long exposure time.

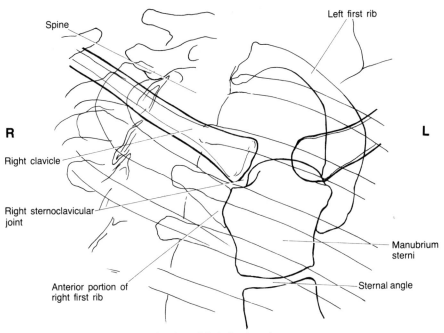

Spine

Left first rib

R

L

Right clavicle

Right sternoclavicular joint

Manubrium sterni

Anterior portion of right first rib

Sternal angle

(Note that the joint nearest to the film is satisfactorily shown)

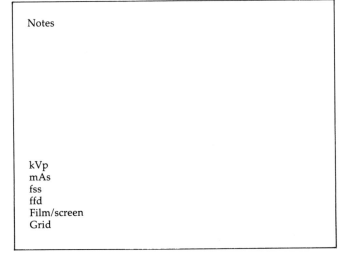

Notes

kVp
mAs
fss
ffd
Film/screen
Grid

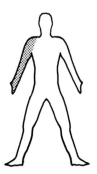

SECTION 2

LOWER LIMB

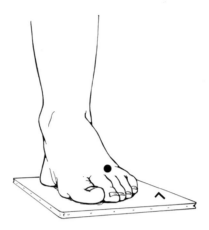

Dorsiplantar (anteroposterior) view of left toes

Equipment required   13 × 18 cm detail screens cassette or non-screen film.
(18 × 24 cm if split and sheet of lead rubber.)
Lead rubber backing sheet for non-screen film.
Lead protective waist apron.

Patient position   Seat the patient on the x-ray couch with the knees flexed. Place plantar aspect of affected foot on film. Support the side under examination with the knee of the other leg to immobilize the foot. Place anatomical marker, collimate beam and apply protection.

Centring point   Head of the third metatarsal or to the individual toe under examination.

Direction of central ray   Vertical at 90° to film.

Special features

L

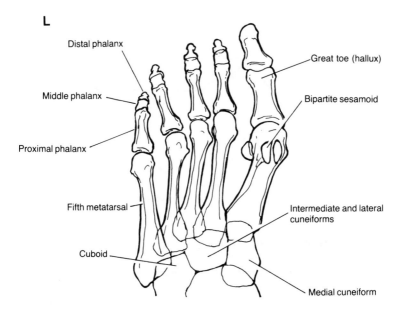

Distal phalanx

Middle phalanx

Proximal phalanx

Fifth metatarsal

Cuboid

Great toe (hallux)

Bipartite sesamoid

Intermediate and lateral cuneiforms

Medial cuneiform

Notes

kVp
mAs
fss
ffd
Film/screen
Grid

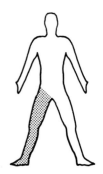

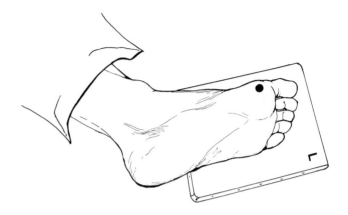

Lateral view of left toes

Equipment required   13 × 18 cm detail screens cassette or
non-screen film.
(18 × 24 cm if split and sheet of lead
rubber.)
Lead rubber backing sheet for
non-screen film.
Large foam pad.
Sandbag.
Lead protective waist apron.

Patient position   Lie the patient on the x-ray couch on the
affected side with the hip and knee flexed. Rest the unaffected
leg in a comfortable position in front of or behind the affected
leg. Place the foot in the true lateral position with the knee
raised on a pad and the film under the toes. Immobilize the
foot. Place anatomical marker, collimate beam, and apply
protection.

Centring point   Head of the first metatarsal.

Direction of central ray   Vertical at 90° to film.

Special features   If a lateral of an individual toe is required
then lie the patient on either side as convenient. Place a dental
film under the toe to be examined which should be as lateral
as possible. The final position will vary according to the
condition of the patient. Centre to the affected toe and ensure
that at least one joint is included.

L

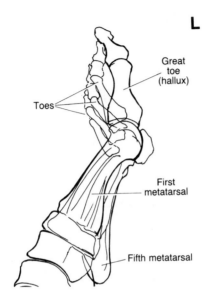

Great
toe
(hallux)

Toes

First
metatarsal

Fifth metatarsal

Notes

kVp
mAs
fss
ffd
Film/screen
Grid

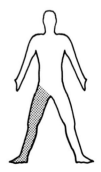

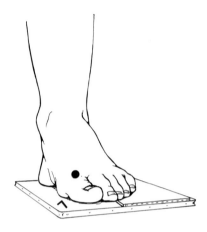

Dorsiplantar (anteroposterior) view of left hallux

Equipment required   13 × 18 cm detail screens cassette or non-screen film.
(18 × 24 cm if split and sheet of lead rubber.)
Lead rubber backing sheet for non-screen film.
Lead protective waist apron.

Patient position   Seat the patient on the x-ray couch with the knees flexed. Place the great toe and sole of affected foot on the film. Support the side under examination with the knee of the other leg to immobilize the foot. Place anatomical marker, collimate beam and apply protection.

Centring point   Head of the first metatarsal.

Direction of central ray   Vertical at 90° to film.

Special features   For hallux valgus the dorsiplantar projection should be used with both feet together weight bearing.

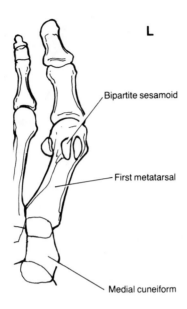

L

Bipartite sesamoid

First metatarsal

Medial cuneiform

Notes

kVp
mAs
fss
ffd
Film/screen
Grid

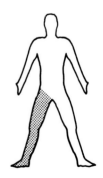

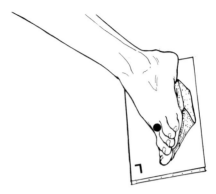

Lateral oblique view of left hallux

Equipment required   13 × 18 cm detail screens cassette or non-screen film.
(18 × 24 cm if split and sheet of lead rubber.)
Lead rubber backing sheet for non-screen film.
Large foam pad or sandbag.
Small foam pad.
Lead protective waist apron.

Patient position   Lie the patient on the unaffected side with the hip and knee of the affected leg slightly flexed. Place the medial aspect of the great toe under examination on the film with the knee resting on a large pad or sandbag. Rotate the foot until the sole of the foot is angled obliquely as shown. Rest the unaffected leg in a comfortable position. Immobilize the foot. Place anatomical marker, collimate beam and apply protection.

Centring point   Head of the first metatarsal.

Direction of central ray   Vertical at 90° to film.

Special features   It is important to avoid superimposing the other toes and metatarsals over the great toe and first metatarsal. If necessary an alternative position may give a more satisfactory projection although this is more difficult for the patient. Further flex the hip of the affected leg with the knee in contact with the couch top. Rotate the foot until the sole of the foot is angled obliquely forwards. Centre over the thenar eminence of the great toe. If required, the sesamoid bones are best demonstrated using the dorsiplantar oblique view of the foot.

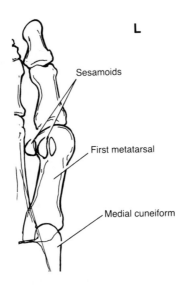

L

Sesamoids

First metatarsal

Medial cuneiform

Notes

kVp
mAs
fss
ffd
Film/screen
Grid

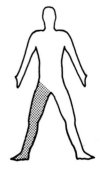

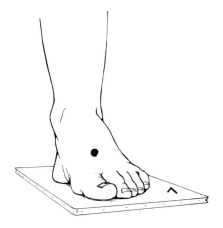

Dorsiplantar (anteroposterior) view of left foot

Equipment required   24 × 30 cm detail screens cassette or
non-screen film (split).
Sheet of lead rubber.
Lead rubber backing sheet for
non-screen film.
Lead protective waist apron.

Patient position   Seat the patient on the x-ray couch with
knees flexed. Place sole of affected foot on film. Support side
under examination with the knee of the other leg to
immobilize the foot and leg. Place anatomical marker,
collimate beam and apply protection.

Centring point   Dorsum of the foot to the cuboid–navicular
region.

Direction of central ray   Vertical at 90° to film.

Special features

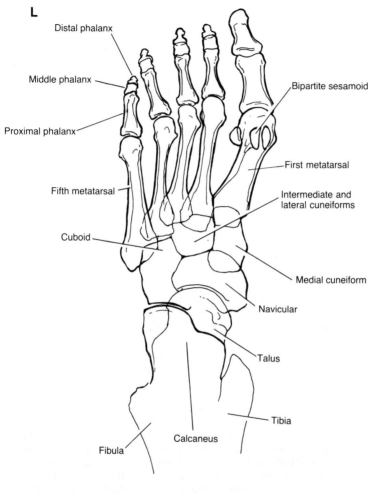

L

Distal phalanx

Middle phalanx

Proximal phalanx

Fifth metatarsal

Cuboid

Bipartite sesamoid

First metatarsal

Intermediate and lateral cuneiforms

Medial cuneiform

Navicular

Talus

Tibia

Calcaneus

Fibula

Notes

kVp
mAs
fss
ffd
Film/screen
Grid

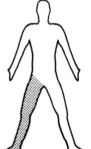

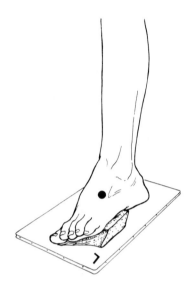

Dorsiplantar oblique view of left foot

Equipment required   24 × 30 cm detail screens cassette or non-screen film (split).
Sheet of lead rubber.
Lead rubber backing sheet for non-screen film.
Small foam pad.
Lead protective waist apron.

Patient position   Seat the patient on the x-ray couch with the knees flexed. Place the affected foot on the film and raise the lateral border on a pad so that the dorsum of the foot is parallel to the film. Support the side under examination with the knee of the other leg to immobilize the foot and leg. Place anatomical marker, collimate beam and apply protection.

Centring point   Dorsum of the foot to the cuboid–navicular region.

Direction of central ray   Vertical at 90° to film.

Special features   The tube may be angled 15° towards the ankle joint in order to show the joint spaces between the tarsal bones more clearly if required.

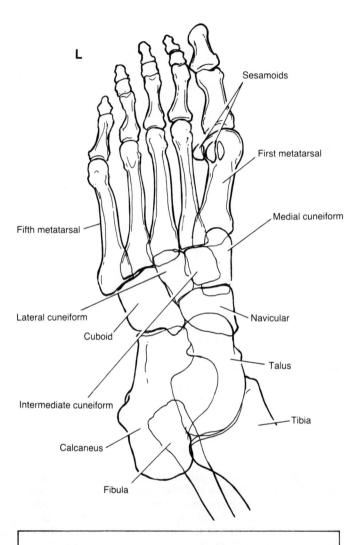

L

Sesamoids

First metatarsal

Medial cuneiform

Fifth metatarsal

Navicular

Lateral cuneiform

Cuboid

Talus

Intermediate cuneiform

Tibia

Calcaneus

Fibula

Notes

kVp
mAs
fss
ffd
Film/screen
Grid

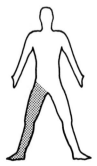

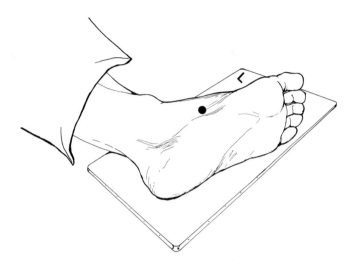

Lateral view of left foot

Equipment required   24 × 30 cm detail screens cassette or non-screen film.
Lead rubber backing sheet for non-screen film.
Large foam pad.
Sandbag.
Lead protective waist apron.

Patient position   Lie the patient on the x-ray couch on the affected side with the hip and knee flexed. Rest the unaffected leg in a comfortable position in front of or behind the affected leg. Raise the knee of the affected leg on a pad and place the foot on the film in the true lateral position. Immobilize the foot. Place anatomical marker, collimate beam and apply protection.

Centring point   Cuboid–navicular area of foot.

Direction of central ray   Vertical at 90° to film.

Special features   This projection is useful for showing the position of foreign bodies or displaced fractured metatarsals.

L

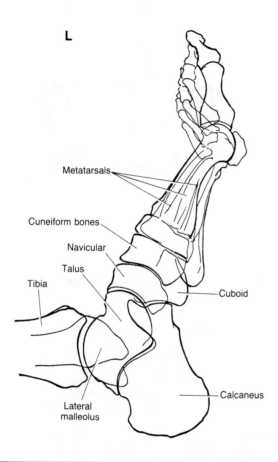

Metatarsals

Cuneiform bones

Navicular

Talus

Tibia

Cuboid

Calcaneus

Lateral
malleolus

Notes

kVp
mAs
fss
ffd
Film/screen
Grid

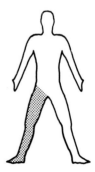

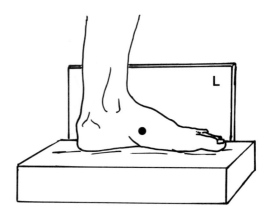

Lateral view of left foot for pes planus (weight bearing)

Equipment required   24 × 30 cm detail screens cassette or non-screen film.
Lead rubber backing sheet for non-screen film.
Block or thick book.
Foam pad or sandbag.
Lead protective waist apron.

Patient position   Stand the patient with the foot under examination on a block in the true lateral position. Support the film vertically with a pad or sandbag against the lateral aspect of the foot. Place the unaffected leg in a comfortable position in front of or behind the affected leg with an equal distribution of weight. Ensure that the patient is well supported. Place anatomical marker, collimate beam and apply protection.

Centring point   Cuboid–navicular area of the foot.

Direction of central ray   Horizontal at 90° to film.

Special features   Both feet are usually examined for comparison.

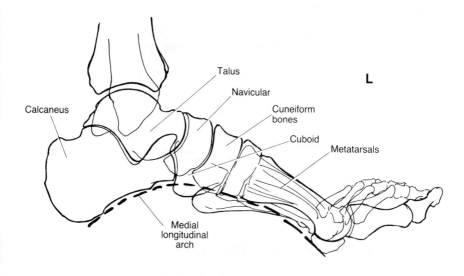

Talus

Navicular

Cuneiform
bones

Cuboid

Metatarsals

Calcaneus

L

Medial
longitudinal
arch

Notes

kVp
mAs
fss
ffd
Film/screen
Grid

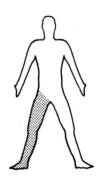

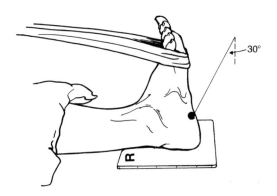

Axial view of right calcaneus

Equipment required   13 × 18 cm detail screens cassette or
non-screen film.
(18 × 24 cm if split and sheet of lead
rubber.)
Lead rubber backing sheet for
non-screen film.
Length of bandage or strong tape.
Sandbag.
Lead protective waist apron.

Patient position   Seat the patient on the x-ray couch with
legs extended and unaffected leg abducted. Dorsiflex the
ankle of the side under examination and place the heel on the
film. Ask the patient to hold the ankle in dorsiflexion with the
bandage or tape. Immobilize the lower leg. Place anatomical
marker, collimate beam and apply protection.

Centring point   Middle of the plantar aspect of the foot.

Direction of central ray   Vertical with tube angled 30° to the
sole of the foot.

Special features   Both heels may need to be examined for
comparison. Extra care should be taken with the dorsiflexion
if a fracture is suspected.

R

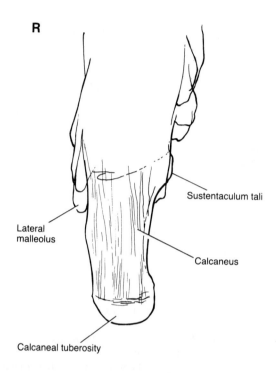

Sustentaculum tali

Lateral
malleolus

Calcaneus

Calcaneal tuberosity

Notes

kVp
mAs
fss
ffd
Film/screen
Grid

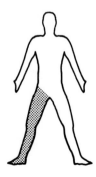

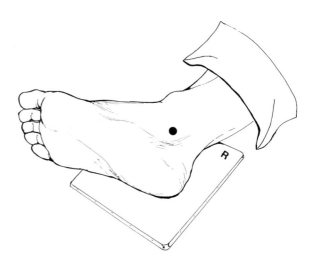

Lateral view of right calcaneus

Equipment required   13 × 18 cm detail screens cassette or non-screen film.
(18 × 24 cm if split and sheet of lead rubber.)
Lead rubber backing sheet for non-screen film.
Large foam pad.
Sandbag.
Lead protective waist apron.

Patient position   Lie the patient on the x-ray couch on the affected side with hip and knee flexed. Rest the unaffected leg in a comfortable position in front of or behind the affected leg. Raise the knee of the affected leg on a pad and place the heel under examination on the film with the foot in the true lateral position. Immobilize the lower leg. Place anatomical marker, collimate beam and apply protection.

Centring point   Talocalcaneal articulation.

Direction of central ray   Vertical at 90° to film.

Special features   Both heels may need to be examined for comparison.

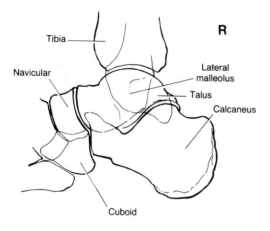

Tibia

Navicular

Lateral
malleolus

Talus

Calcaneus

R

Cuboid

Notes

kVp
mAs
fss
ffd
Film/screen
Grid

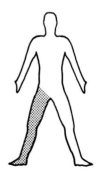

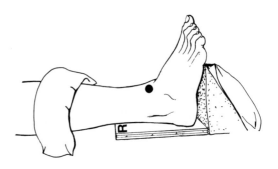

Anteroposterior view of right ankle

Equipment required   18 × 24 cm detail screens cassette or non-screen film.
(24 × 30 cm if split and sheet of lead rubber.)
Lead rubber backing sheet for non-screen film.
Foam pad.
Sandbag.
Lead protective waist apron.

Patient position   Seat the patient on the x-ray couch with the legs extended and unaffected leg abducted. Place the ankle under examination on the cassette or film with the joint flexed at 90°. Rotate the ankle medially until both malleoli are equidistant from the couch top. Immobilize the lower leg by supporting the sole of the foot with a pad and sandbag. Place anatomical marker, collimate beam and apply protection.

Centring point   Midway between the malleoli.

Direction of central ray   Vertical at 90° to the film.

Special features   An additional modified anteroposterior projection with forced inversion may be required to demonstrate damaged lateral ligaments. This has the effect of widening the lateral aspect of the joint space. A routine anteroposterior view should be taken first to exclude bony injury. The forced inversion must only be carried out by a medical officer suitably protected with a lead protective apron and lead rubber gloves.

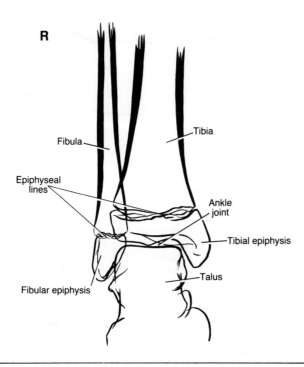

R

Fibula

Tibia

Epiphyseal
lines

Ankle
joint

Tibial epiphysis

Talus

Fibular epiphysis

Notes

kVp
mAs
fss
ffd
Film/screen
Grid

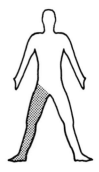

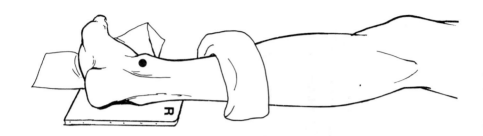

Lateral view of right ankle

Equipment required   18 × 24 cm detail screens cassette or non-screen film.
(24 × 30 cm if split and sheet of lead rubber.)
Lead rubber backing sheet for non-screen film.
Foam pad.
Sandbag.
Lead protective waist apron.

Patient position   Lie the patient on the affected side with hip and knee flexed. Rest the unaffected leg in a comfortable position in front of or behind the affected leg. Raise the knee of the affected leg on a pad and place the lateral aspect of the ankle under examination on the film with the joint flexed at 90°. Rotate the ankle laterally until the malleoli are superimposed. Support the raised foot with a pad under the toes. Immobilize the lower leg. Place anatomical marker, collimate beam and apply protection.

Centring point   Medial malleolus.

Direction of central ray   Vertical at 90° to film.

Special features   To demonstrate the subtalar joint keep the foot in the true lateral position.

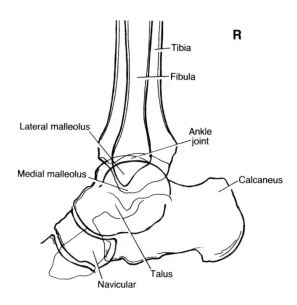

R

Tibia

Fibula

Lateral malleolus

Ankle joint

Medial malleolus

Calcaneus

Navicular

Talus

Notes

kVp
mAs
fss
ffd
Film/screen
Grid

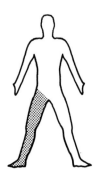

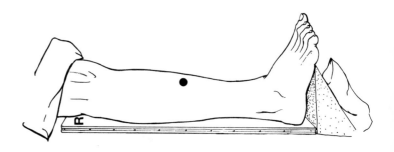

Anteroposterior view of right tibia and fibula

Equipment required   35 × 43 cm detail screens cassette (split).
Sheet of lead rubber.
Foam pad.
Sandbag.
Lead protective waist apron.

Patient position   Lie the patient on the x-ray couch with legs extended and unaffected leg abducted. Place the lower leg under examination on the cassette and flex the ankle at 90° with the foot upright. Include both the ankle and knee joints on the film if possible. Immobilize the leg by supporting the sole of the foot with a pad and sandbag. Place anatomical marker, collimate beam and apply protection.

Centring point   Anterior aspect of the middle of the lower leg midway between the ankle and knee.

Direction of central ray   Vertical at 90° to the film.

Special features   It is important to include both joints on the film in cases of trauma since a fracture of the lower tibia and fibula may be accompanied by a fracture in the region of the upper fibula.

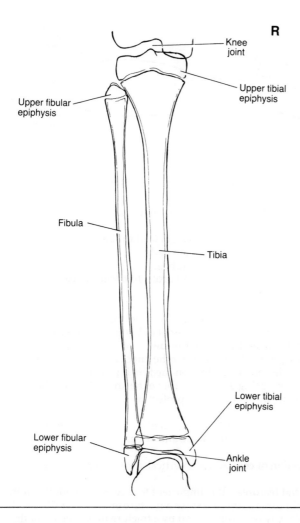

R

Knee joint

Upper tibial epiphysis

Upper fibular epiphysis

Fibula

Tibia

Lower tibial epiphysis

Lower fibular epiphysis

Ankle joint

Notes

kVp
mAs
fss
ffd
Film/screen
Grid

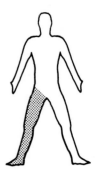

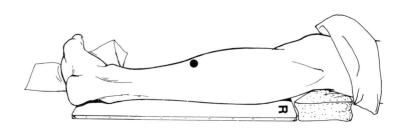

Lateral view of right tibia and fibula

Equipment required   35 × 43 cm detail screens cassette (split).
Sheet of lead rubber.
Foam pads.
Sandbag.
Lead protective waist apron.

Patient position   Lie the patient on the affected side with the hip and knee slightly flexed. Rest the unaffected leg in a comfortable position in front of or behind the affected leg. Place the lateral aspect of the lower leg under examination on the cassette with pads under the knee and toes. Include both the ankle and knee joints on the film if possible. Immobilize the leg by using a sandbag above the knee. Place marker, collimate beam and apply protection.

Centring point   Medial aspect of the middle of the lower leg, midway between the ankle and knee.

Direction of central ray   Vertical at 90° to film.

Special features   It is important to include both joints on the film in cases of trauma since a fracture of the lower tibia and fibula may be accompanied by a fracture in the region of the upper fibula.

Important note   A horizontal lateral projection should be used if the patient cannot be turned due to severe injury.

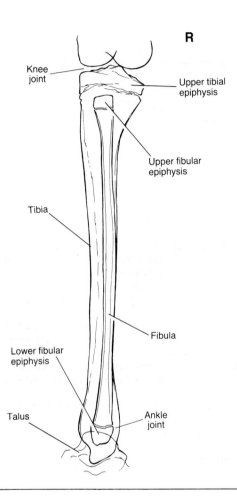

R

Knee joint

Upper tibial epiphysis

Upper fibular epiphysis

Tibia

Fibula

Lower fibular epiphysis

Talus

Ankle joint

Notes

kVp
mAs
fss
ffd
Film/screen
Grid

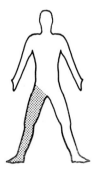

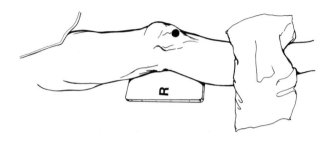

Anteroposterior view of right knee

Equipment required   18 × 24 cm detail screens cassette.
(24 × 30 cm if split and sheet of lead
rubber.)
Sandbag.
Lead protective waist apron.

Patient position   Lie the patient on the x-ray couch with legs
extended and unaffected leg abducted. Place the knee under
examination on the film and flex the joint slightly. Ensure that
the patella is central over the femur. Immobilize the leg. Place
anatomical marker, collimate beam and apply protection.

Centring point   2.5 cm below the apex of the patella.

Direction of central ray   Vertical at 90° to film.

Special features

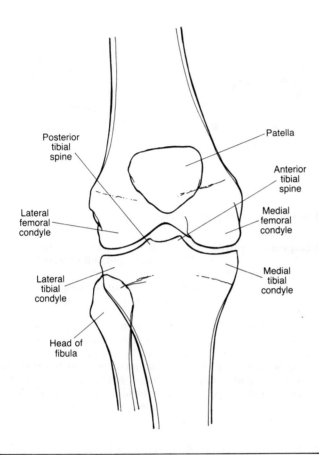

Posterior
tibial
spine

Patella

Anterior
tibial
spine

Lateral
femoral
condyle

Medial
femoral
condyle

Lateral
tibial
condyle

Medial
tibial
condyle

Head of
fibula

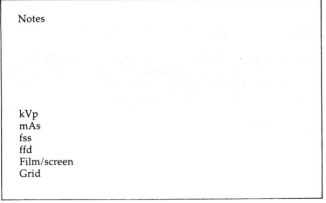

Notes

kVp
mAs
fss
ffd
Film/screen
Grid

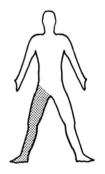

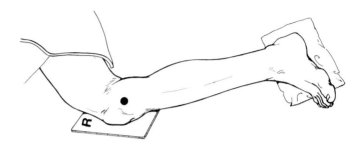

Lateral view of right knee

Equipment required   18 × 24 cm detail screens cassette.
(24 × 30 cm if split and sheet of lead rubber.)
Large foam pad or sandbag.
Lead protective waist apron.

Patient position   Lie the patient on the affected side with hip and knee flexed. Rest the unaffected leg in a comfortable position preferably in front of the affected leg. Place the lateral aspect of the knee under examination on the film. Support the ankle with a pad or sandbag. Ensure that the tibia is parallel and the patella perpendicular to the film. Immobilize the leg. Place anatomical marker, collimate beam and apply protection.

Centring point   Anterior border of the medial condyle of the tibia.

Direction of central ray   Vertical at 90° to film.

Special features   The tube may be angled 5° towards the head (cephalic) in order to superimpose the condyles of the femur. If the tibial tubercle is required then laterals of both knees may be taken for comparison to demonstrate osteochondritis (Osgood–Schlatter's disease). Centre over the tibial tubercle. Reduce the tube kilovoltage and closely collimate beam.

R

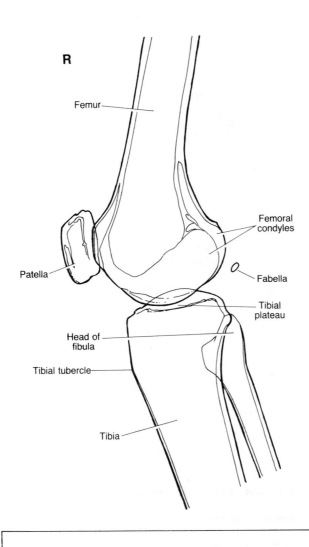

Femur

Femoral condyles

Patella

Fabella

Tibial plateau

Head of fibula

Tibial tubercle

Tibia

Notes

kVp
mAs
fss
ffd
Film/screen
Grid

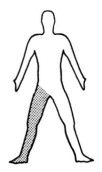

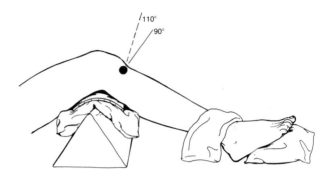

Modified anteroposterior (tunnel) views of right knee for intercondylar notch

Equipment required   Two 18 × 24 cm detail screens curved cassettes if available, or flexible non-screen films.
Lead rubber backing sheet for non-screen film.
Sandbags.
Large foam pads.
Lead protective waist apron.

Patient position   Seat the patient on the x-ray couch. Flex the knee and rest on the cassette or film supported by a sandbag and pad as required. Abduct the other leg and rest in a comfortable position. Immobilize the knee. Place anatomical marker, collimate beam and apply protection.

Centring point   Apex of the patella.

Direction of central ray

Projection 1   90° to the shaft of the tibia.

Projection 2   110° to the shaft of the tibia.

Special features   Projection 1 demonstrates the posterior aspect of the intercondylar notch. Projection 2 demonstrates the anterior aspect.

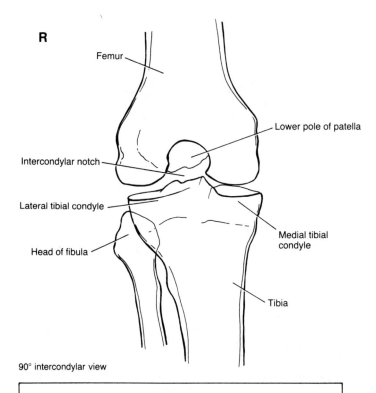

R

Femur

Lower pole of patella

Intercondylar notch

Lateral tibial condyle

Medial tibial condyle

Head of fibula

Tibia

90° intercondylar view

Notes

kVp
mAs
fss
ffd
Film/screen
Grid

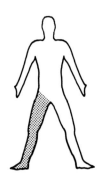

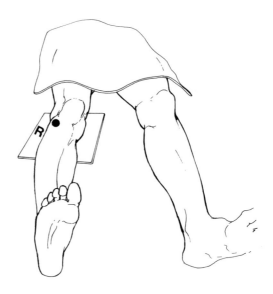

Anteroposterior oblique view of right superior tibiofibular joint

Equipment required   18 × 24 cm detail screens cassette or non-screen film.
Lead rubber backing sheet for non-screen film.
Lead protective waist apron.

Patient position   Seat the patient on the x-ray couch with legs extended and the unaffected leg abducted. Place the knee of the leg under examination on the film. Rotate the leg medially until the head of the fibula is in profile. Immobilize the leg. Place anatomical marker, collimate beam and apply protection.

Centring point   Superior tibiofibular joint.

Direction of central ray   Vertical at 90° to the film.

Special features

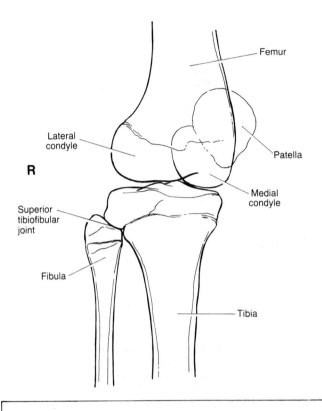

Femur

Lateral
condyle

Patella

R

Medial
condyle

Superior
tibiofibular
joint

Fibula

Tibia

Notes

kVp
mAs
fss
ffd
Film/screen
Grid

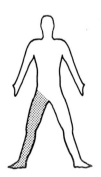

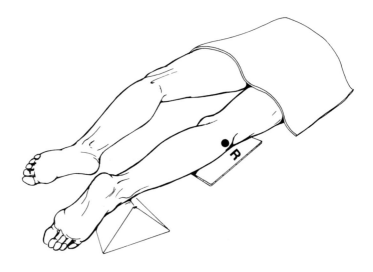

Lateral oblique view of right superior tibiofibular joint

Equipment required   18 × 24 cm detail screens cassette or non-screen film.
Lead rubber backing sheet for non-screen film.
Large foam pad.
Lead protective waist apron.

Patient position   Lie the patient prone on the x-ray couch with legs extended. Rest the unaffected leg in a comfortable position with the hip and knee flexed. Place the knee of the leg under examination on the film. Rotate the patient towards the affected side until the head of the fibula is in profile. Support the ankle on a pad and immobilize the leg. Place anatomical marker, collimate beam and apply protection.

Centring point   Superior tibiofibular joint.

Direction of central ray   Vertical at 90° to the film.

Special features

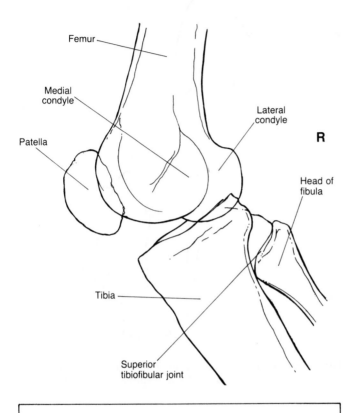

Femur

Medial
condyle

Lateral
condyle

R

Patella

Head of
fibula

Tibia

Superior
tibiofibular joint

Notes

kVp
mAs
fss
ffd
Film/screen
Grid

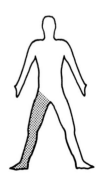

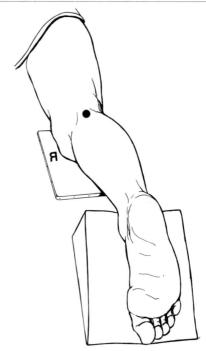

Posteroanterior view of right patella

Equipment required   18 × 24 cm detail screens cassette.
(24 × 30 cm if split and sheet of lead
rubber.)
Foam pad.
Lead protective waist apron.

Patient position   Lie the patient prone on the x-ray couch
with legs extended. Abduct the unaffected leg and rest in a
comfortable position. Place anterior aspect of the patella
under examination on the cassette and flex the knee slightly.
Immobilize the leg by supporting the ankle on a pad. Place
anatomical marker, collimate beam and apply protection.

Centring point   In the midline to the skin crease behind the
knee.

Direction of central ray   Vertical at 90° to the film.

Special features   The tube kilovoltage should be increased
by 10–15 kVp compared with an anteroposterior knee.

Important note   If a fractured patella is suspected the knee
should *not* be flexed. An anteroposterior projection should be
used with the patient kept supine.

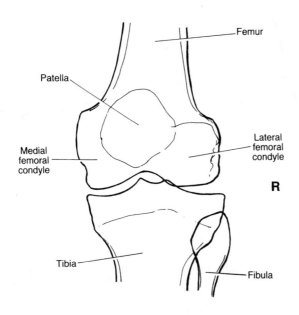

Femur

Patella

Medial
femoral
condyle

Lateral
femoral
condyle

R

Tibia

Fibula

Notes

kVp
mAs
fss
ffd
Film/screen
Grid

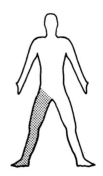

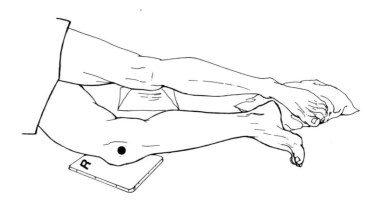

Lateral view of right patella

Equipment required   10 × 24 cm detail screens cassette.
(24 × 30 cm if split and sheet of lead rubber.)
Large foam pad.
Sandbag.
Lead protective waist apron.

Patient position   Lie the patient on the x-ray couch on the affected side with hip and knee flexed. Support the unaffected leg in a comfortable position behind the affected leg with a pad or sandbag. Place the lateral aspect of the knee under examination on the cassette and ensure that the patella is in the true lateral position. Immobilize the leg. Place anatomical marker, collimate beam and apply protection.

Centring point   Medial aspect of patella.

Direction of central ray   Vertical at 90° to film.

Special features

Important note   If a fractured patella is suspected the knee should *not* be flexed. A horizontal beam lateral projection should be used with the patient kept supine.

R

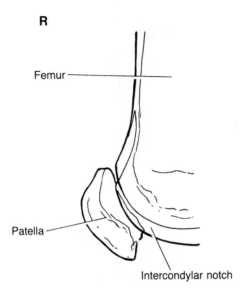

Femur

Patella

Intercondylar notch

Notes

kVp
mAs
fss
ffd
Film/screen
Grid

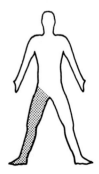

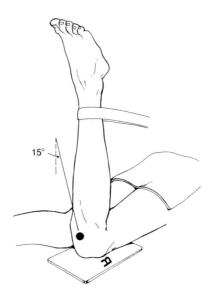

Inferosuperior view of right patella

Equipment required   18 × 24 cm detail screens cassette.
Short length of bandage.
Large foam pad.
Sandbag.
Lead protective waist apron.

Patient position   Lie the patient prone on the x-ray couch.
Rest the unaffected leg in a comfortable position with a
sandbag or pad under the ankle. Flex the knee of the affected
leg at 90° with the foot extended. Immobilize the leg by
supporting it in flexion with the bandage looped around the
ankle and held by the patient. Place anatomical marker,
collimate beam and apply protection.

Centring point   Behind the apex of the patella.

Direction of central ray   Vertical with tube angled 15°
towards the head (cephalic).

Special features   This projection should not be used if a
fracture of the patella is suspected.

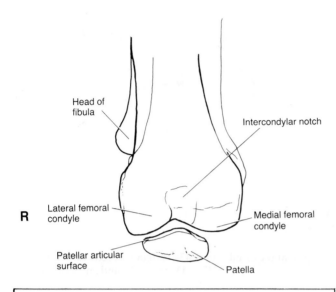

Head of fibula

Intercondylar notch

R

Lateral femoral condyle

Medial femoral condyle

Patellar articular surface

Patella

Notes

kVp
mAs
fss
ffd
Film/screen
Grid

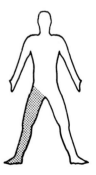

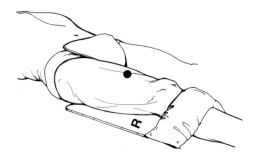

Anteroposterior view of right femur — lower two-thirds

Equipment required   18 × 43 cm detail screens cassette. (35 × 43 cm if split and sheet of lead rubber.)
Foam pad.
Lead rubber gonad protection.

Patient position   Lie the patient supine with both legs extended, abduct the unaffected leg and rest in a comfortable position. Include the knee joint of the leg under examination. Immobilize the lower leg with a sandbag. Place anatomical marker, collimate beam and apply protection.

Centring point   Anterior aspect of the thigh to the middle of the film.

Direction of central ray   Vertical at 90° to film.

Special features

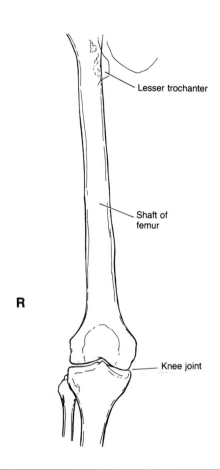

Lesser trochanter

Shaft of
femur

R

Knee joint

Notes

kVp
mAs
fss
ffd
Film/screen
Grid

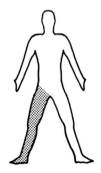

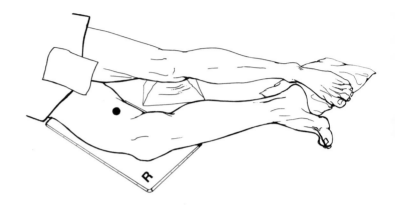

Lateral view of right femur — lower two-thirds

Equipment required   18 × 43 cm detail screens cassette.
(35 × 43 cm if split and sheet of lead
rubber).
Foam pad.
Sandbag.
Lead rubber gonad protection.

Patient position   Lie the patient on the affected side with the
hip and knee flexed. Rest the unaffected leg in a comfortable
position behind the affected leg. Place the lateral aspect of the
leg under examination on the film with a pad under the ankle.
Include the knee joint. Immobilize the lower leg with a
sandbag. Place anatomical marker, collimate beam and apply
protection.

Centring point   Medial aspect of the thigh to the middle of
the film.

Direction of central ray   Vertical at 90° to film.

Special features   In cases of severe injury, if this projection is
impracticable, then lie the patient supine and raise and
support the unaffected limb. Place the film against the lateral
aspect of the leg under examination and use a horizontal
beam.

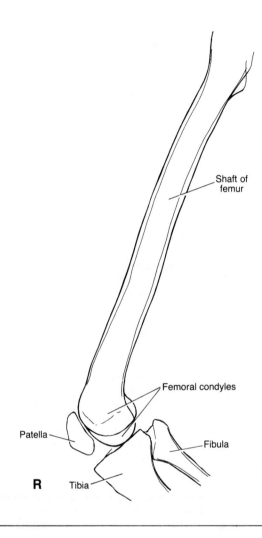

Shaft of
femur

Femoral condyles

Patella

Fibula

R

Tibia

Notes

kVp
mAs
fss
ffd
Film/screen
Grid

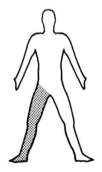

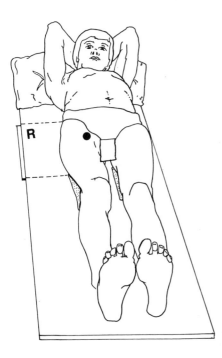

Centring point

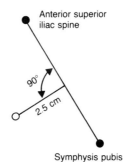

Anterior superior
iliac spine

90°

2.5 cm

Symphysis pubis

Anteroposterior view of right hip joint and upper third of femur

Equipment required
24 × 30 cm detail or fast screens cassette.
Table bucky or stationary grid or
gridded cassette.
Foam pads.
Lead rubber gonad protection.

Patient position   Lie the patient supine with the hip under
examination in the centre of the x-ray couch. Extend both legs,
flex knees slightly and rest on pads. Ensure that the trunk is
not rotated and that the pelvis is level. Rotate both legs
medially and place great toes together with heels apart if
possible. Rest the hands above the head or on the chest.
Immobilize the patient. Place anatomical marker, collimate
beam and apply gonad protection if possible without
obscuring the hip joint.

Centring point   To the hip joint at a point 2.5 cm distal along
the perpendicular bisection of a line from the anterior
superior iliac spine to the upper border of the symphysis
pubis.

Direction of central ray   Vertical at 90° to film.

Special features   Expose on arrested respiration. In the event
of trauma the initial examination should include the whole
pelvis and gonad protection may be omitted. If there is
obvious external rotation of the injured limb, then medial
rotation should *not* be attempted since this is an indication of
a fractured neck of femur.

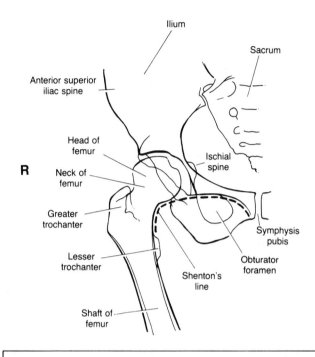

Ilium

Sacrum

Anterior superior
iliac spine

Head of
femur

Ischial
spine

R

Neck of
femur

Greater
trochanter

Symphysis
pubis

Lesser
trochanter

Obturator
foramen

Shenton's
line

Shaft of
femur

Notes

kVp
mAs
fss
ffd
Film/screen
Grid

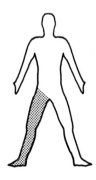

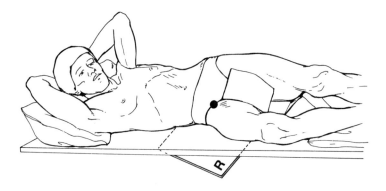

Lateral view of right hip joint and upper third of femur

Equipment required   24 × 30 cm detail or fast screens cassette (or gridded cassette). Table bucky or stationary grid. Foam pads. Sandbags. Lead rubber gonad protection.

Patient position   Lie the patient on the affected side in the centre of the x-ray couch in the true lateral position with the hip and knees flexed. Rotate the patient backwards until the pelvis is at 45° and support. Rest the unaffected leg behind in a comfortable position. Rest the arms in a comfortable position away from the film. Immobilize the patient. Place anatomical marker, collimate beam and apply protection if possible without obscuring the hip joint.

Centring point   To the hip joint just below the crease of the groin in the midline of the thigh.

Direction of central ray   Vertical at 90° to film.

Special features   Place the film obliquely so that the long axis is in line with the shaft of the femur of the side under examination. Expose on arrested respiration. Gonad protection may not be used for the initial examination in cases of injury.

Important note   A horizontal lateral projection should be used if the patient cannot be turned because of severe injury.

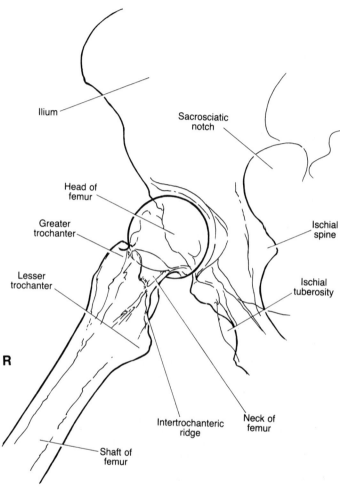

Ilium

Sacrosciatic
notch

Head of
femur

Greater
trochanter

Ischial
spine

Lesser
trochanter

Ischial
tuberosity

R

Intertrochanteric
ridge

Neck of
femur

Shaft of
femur

Notes

kVp
mAs
fss
ffd
Film/screen
Grid

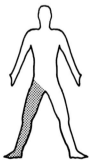

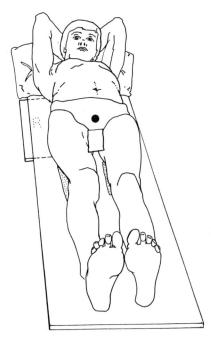

Anteroposterior view of both hip joints

Equipment required
35 × 43 cm detail or fast screens cassette.
Table bucky or stationary grid or
gridded cassette.
Foam pads.
Lead rubber gonad protection.

Patient position   Lie the patient supine in the centre of the
x-ray couch with both legs extended and knees slightly flexed
on pads. Ensure that the trunk is not rotated and that the
pelvis is level. Rotate both legs medially and place the great
toes together with the heels apart if possible. Rest the hands
above the head or on the chest. Immobilize the patient. Place
anatomical marker, collimate beam and apply gonad
protection if possible without obscuring the hip joints.

Centring point   In the midline 2.5 cm above the upper border
of the symphysis pubis.

Direction of central ray   Vertical at 90° to film.

Special features   Place the film transversely with upper edge
just below the iliac crest. In the event of trauma gonad
protection may be omitted. If there is obvious external
rotation of an injured limb, then medial rotation should *not* be
attempted, since this is an indication of a fractured neck of
femur. The sound limb should be rotated to a similar position
for comparison.

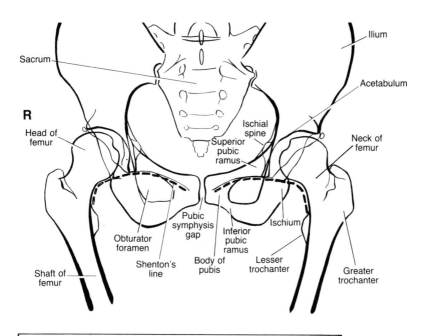

Ilium

Sacrum

Acetabulum

R

Head of
femur

Ischial
spine

Superior
pubic
ramus

Neck of
femur

Pubic
symphysis
gap

Obturator
foramen

Inferior
pubic
ramus

Ischium

Shenton's
line

Body of
pubis

Lesser
trochanter

Greater
trochanter

Shaft of
femur

Notes

kVp
mAs
fss
ffd
Film/screen
Grid

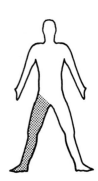

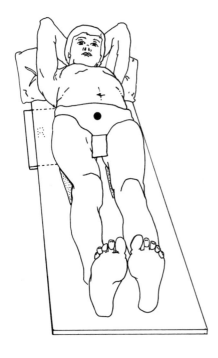

Anteroposterior view of pelvis

Equipment required
35 × 43 cm detail or fast screens cassette.
Table bucky or stationary grid or
gridded cassette.
Foam pads.
Lead rubber gonad protection.

Patient position　Lie the patient supine in the centre of the
x-ray couch with both legs extended and knees slightly flexed
on pads. Ensure that the trunk is not rotated and that the
pelvis is level (symmetrical). Rotate both legs medially and
place the great toes together with heels apart if possible. Rest
the hands above the head or on the chest. Immobilize the
patient. Place anatomical marker, collimate beam and apply
gonad protection if possible without obscuring the pelvis.

Centring point　In the midline 5 cm above the upper border
of the symphysis pubis.

Direction of central ray　Vertical at 90° to the film.

Special features　Place the film transversely to include the
iliac crests. Expose on arrested respiration. In the event of
trauma, gonad protection may be omitted. If there is obvious
external rotation of an injured limb, then medial rotation
should *not* be attempted since this is an indication of a
fractured neck of femur.

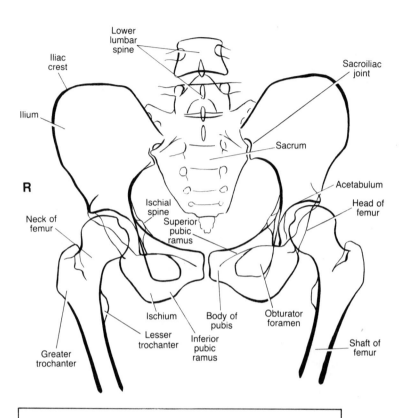

Lower lumbar spine

Iliac crest

Ilium

Sacroiliac joint

Sacrum

R

Acetabulum

Head of femur

Ischial spine

Neck of femur

Superior pubic ramus

Ischium

Body of pubis

Obturator foramen

Lesser trochanter

Inferior pubic ramus

Greater trochanter

Shaft of femur

Notes

kVp
mAs
fss
ffd
Film/screen
Grid

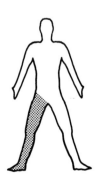

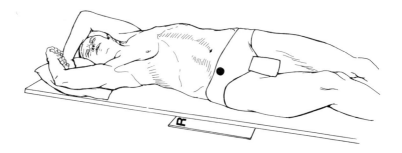

Posterior oblique view of pelvis for right ilium

Equipment required   30 × 40 cm detail or fast screens
cassette.
Table bucky or stationary grid or
gridded cassette.
Foam pads.
Sandbags.
Lead rubber gonad protection.

Patient position   Lie the patient supine with the affected side
in the centre of the x-ray couch and with the legs extended.
Rotate the patient about 30° towards the side under
examination to bring the iliac fossa parallel to the couch top.
Support the raised side on pads. Ensure that the iliac crest is
included on the film. Flex the hip and knee of the affected side
and rest the other leg behind in a comfortable position. Place
the arms in a comfortable position away from the film.
Immobilize the patient by using pads and sandbags. Place
anatomical marker, collimate beam and apply gonad
protection if possible without obscuring the pelvis.

Centring point   To the iliac fossa on the affected side
midway between the anterior superior iliac spine and the
midline.

Direction of central ray   Vertical at 90° to film.

Special features   Expose on arrested respiration. If a fracture
of the pelvis is suspected then this projection should be used
with caution and only if the condition of the patient permits.

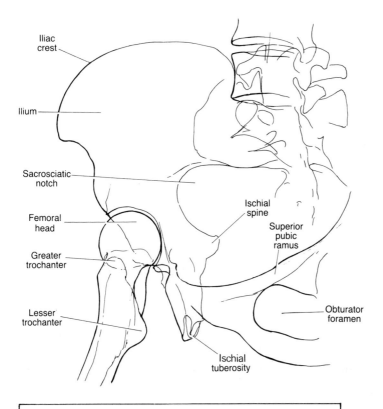

Iliac crest

Ilium

Sacrosciatic notch

Femoral head

Greater trochanter

Lesser trochanter

Ischial spine

Superior pubic ramus

Obturator foramen

Ischial tuberosity

Notes

kVp
mAs
fss
ffd
Film/screen
Grid

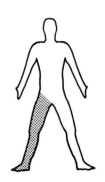

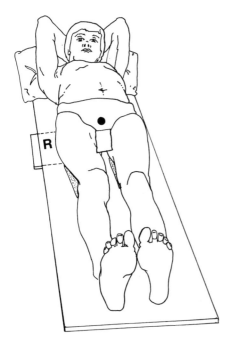

Anteroposterior view of symphysis pubis

Equipment required
24 × 30 cm detail or fast screens cassette (or gridded cassette).
Table bucky or stationary grid.
Foam pads.
Lead rubber gonad protection.

Patient position   Lie the patient supine in the centre of the couch with legs extended and knees slightly flexed on pads. Ensure that the trunk is not rotated and that the pelvis is level. Rest the hands on the chest or above the head. Immobilize the patient. Place anatomical marker, collimate beam and apply protection if possible taking great care not to obscure the symphysis pubis especially in female patients.

Centring point   In the midline to the symphysis pubis.

Direction of central ray   Vertical with tube angled 5° towards the head (cephalic).

Special features   Expose on arrested respiration. If a subluxation is suspected then two projections may be taken with the patient in the erect position with the body weight first on one foot and then on the other. Either anteroposterior or posteroanterior views may be used.

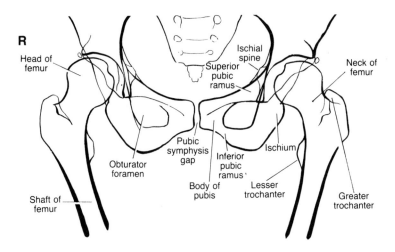

R

Head of femur

Ischial spine

Superior pubic ramus

Neck of femur

Pubic symphysis gap

Inferior pubic ramus

Ischium

Obturator foramen

Body of pubis

Lesser trochanter

Shaft of femur

Greater trochanter

Notes

kVp
mAs
fss
ffd
Film/screen
Grid

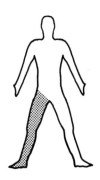

SECTION 3

VERTEBRAL COLUMN

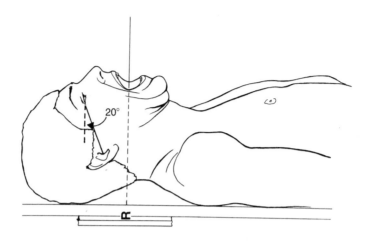

Anteroposterior open mouth view of cervical
vertebrae 1–3

Equipment required   18 × 24 cm detail screens cassette.
Table bucky.
Foam pads.
Sandbags.
Lead protective waist apron.

Patient position   Lie the patient supine in the centre of the
x-ray couch. Rest the back of the head on the couch top and
ensure that the head is not rotated. Extend the neck until the
radiographic baseline is at 20° from the vertical. Immobilize
the head in this position and open the mouth as fully as
possible. Place anatomical marker, collimate beam and apply
protection.

Centring point   To centre of open mouth.

Direction of central ray   Vertical at 90° to the film and parallel
to the hard palate.

Special features   A radiolucent bite block may be used to
keep the mouth open if necessary. Expose during arrested
respiration. The patient may also be examined in the erect
position using a vertical bucky. A grid is not essential for
either position. The pads and sandbags used for
immobilization are not shown to avoid obscuring the position
of the head.

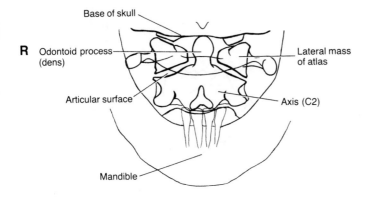

R

Base of skull

Odontoid process (dens)

Lateral mass of atlas

Articular surface

Axis (C2)

Mandible

Notes

kVp
mAs
fss
ffd
Film/screen
Grid

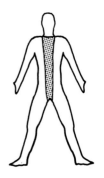

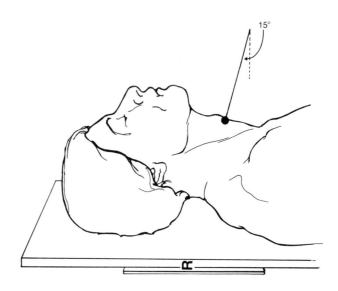

Anteroposterior view of cervical vertebrae 3–7

Equipment required   24 × 30 cm detail screens cassette.
Table bucky.
Foam pads.
Sandbags.
Lead protective rubber apron.

Patient position   Lie the patient supine in the centre of the
x-ray couch. Rest back of the head on the couch top and
ensure that the head is not rotated. Raise the chin until the
lower border of the mandible is at 90° to the film. Immobilize
the head in this position. Place anatomical marker, collimate
beam and apply protection.

Centring point   In the midline 5 cm above the suprasternal
notch.

Direction of central ray   Vertical with the tube angled 15°
towards the head (cephalad).

Special features   Expose during arrested respiration. The
patient may also be examined in the erect position using the
vertical bucky. A grid is not essential for either position. The
pads and sandbags used for immobilization are not shown, to
avoid obscuring the position of the head.

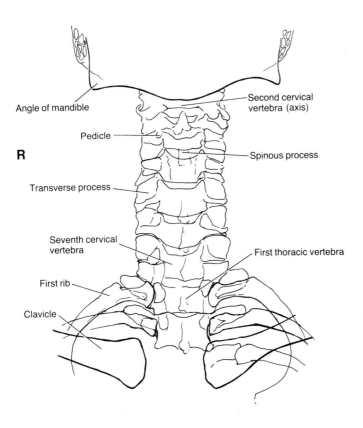

Angle of mandible

Second cervical vertebra (axis)

Pedicle

Spinous process

R

Transverse process

Seventh cervical vertebra

First thoracic vertebra

First rib

Clavicle

Notes

kVp
mAs
fss
ffd
Film/screen
Grid

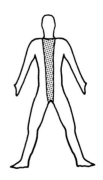

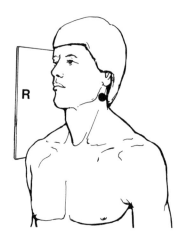

Right lateral view of cervical spine

Equipment required   24 × 30 cm detail screens cassette.
Erect cassette holder.
Foam pads.
Lead protective waist apron.

Patient position   Stand or sit the patient in the true lateral
position against the erect cassette holder. Raise the chin until
the angle of the mandible is clear of the cervical vertebrae.
Depress the shoulders as low as possible. Rest the tip of the
shoulder on the lower border of the cassette. Immobilize the
head with foam pads if necessary. Place anatomical marker,
collimate beam and apply protection.

Centring point   2.5 cm posterior to the angle of the mandible.

Direction of central ray   Horizontal at 90° to the film.

Special features   Use a focus–film distance of at least 150 cm
to compensate for the very large object–film distance. Expose
during arrested respiration. The arms may need to be weight
bearing in order to demonstrate the seventh cervical vertebra.
In cases of severe injury the patient should be examined in the
supine position using a horizontal lateral projection.

Important note   Flexion and extension lateral views may be
required to demonstrate instability of the cervical spine, but
these should only be taken after the routine projections and in
the presence of a medical officer.

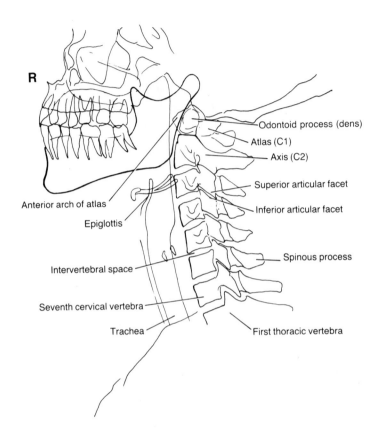

R

Odontoid process (dens)
Atlas (C1)
Axis (C2)
Superior articular facet
Inferior articular facet
Anterior arch of atlas
Epiglottis
Spinous process
Intervertebral space
Seventh cervical vertebra
Trachea
First thoracic vertebra

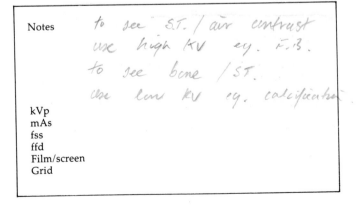

Notes   to see S.T. / air contrast
use high KV eg. F.B.
to see bone / ST.
use low KV eg. calcification

kVp
mAs
fss
ffd
Film/screen
Grid

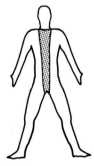

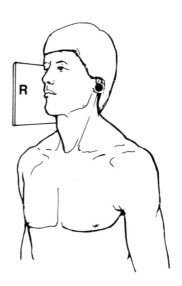

Right lateral view of cervical spine for atlanto-occipital articulation

Equipment required   18 × 24 cm detail screens cassette.
Vertical cassette holder.
Small localizing cone.
Lead protective waist apron.

Patient position   Stand or sit the patient in the true lateral position against the vertical cassette holder. Place the head and neck in contact with the cassette. Immobilize the head. Place anatomical marker, collimate beam using a small localizing cone and apply protection.

Centring point   2.5 cm below and behind the external auditory meatus.

Direction of central ray   Horizontal at 90° to the film.

Special features   Expose on arrested respiration. The patient may be examined supine instead of in the erect position if preferred.

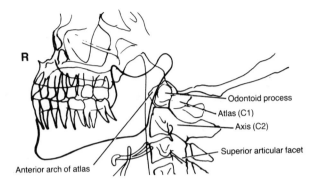

R

Odontoid process
Atlas (C1)
Axis (C2)
Superior articular facet

Anterior arch of atlas

Notes

kVp
mAs
fss
ffd
Film/screen
Grid

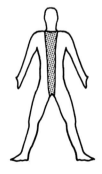

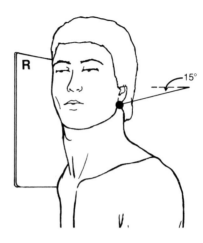

Right anterior oblique view of cervical spine

SHOWS ⓇINTERVERTEBRAL FORAMINA ✗

Equipment required 24 × 30 cm detail screens cassette.
Vertical bucky.
Foam pads.
Lead protective waist apron.

Patient position Stand or sit the patient facing the vertical
bucky stand with the neck in the centre. Rotate the patient 45°
to the left and right sides in turn. Depress the chin slightly
and turn the head until the median sagittal plane is parallel to
the film. Immobilize the patient using foam pads if necessary.
Place anatomical marker, collimate beam and apply
protection.

Centring point To the middle of the neck, 2.5 cm below the
angle of the mandible on the side nearest the film.

Direction of central ray Horizontal with tube angled 15°
towards the feet (caudad).

Special features Expose on arrested respiration. Both sides
are usually taken for comparison. The intervertebral foramina
nearest to the film are demonstrated. As an alternative the
patient may be examined facing the x-ray tube for the right
and left posterior oblique projections. The central ray is
angled 15° towards the head (cephalad). The intervertebral
foramina remote from the film are demonstrated. If the
intervertebral facets are required then the patient should only
be rotated 28°.

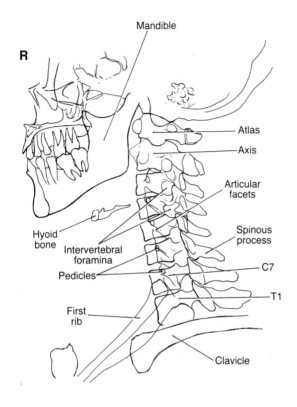

R

Mandible

Atlas

Axis

Articular
facets

Spinous
process

Hyoid
bone

Intervertebral
foramina

Pedicles

C7

T1

First
rib

Clavicle

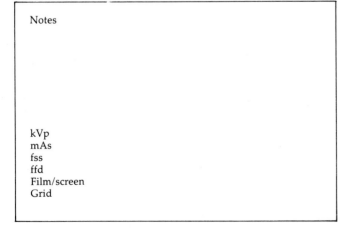

Notes

kVp
mAs
fss
ffd
Film/screen
Grid

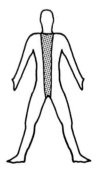

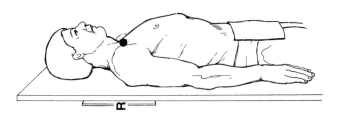

Anteroposterior view of cervicothoracic spine

Equipment required   24 × 30 cm detail screens cassette.
Table bucky.
Lead protective waist apron.

Patient position   Lie the patient supine in the centre of the
x-ray couch with the hands and arms to the side of the body.
Raise the chin slightly and ensure that the head is not rotated.
Include the fourth cervical to the fourth thoracic vertebrae on
the film. Immobilize the patient. Place anatomical marker,
collimate beam and apply protection.

Centring point   Suprasternal notch.

Direction of central ray   Vertical at 90° to the film.

Special features   Expose on arrested respiration. The patient
may be examined in the erect position using the vertical
bucky.

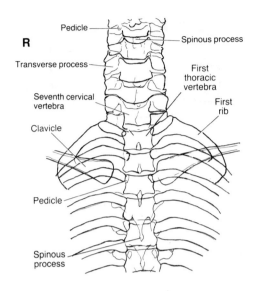

R

Pedicle

Spinous process

Transverse process

First thoracic vertebra

Seventh cervical vertebra

First rib

Clavicle

Pedicle

Spinous process

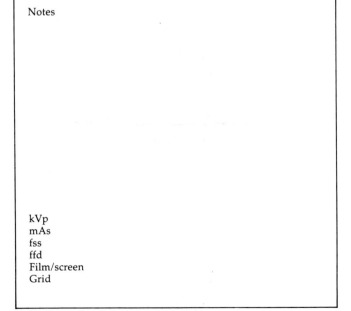

Notes

kVp
mAs
fss
ffd
Film/screen
Grid

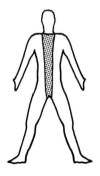

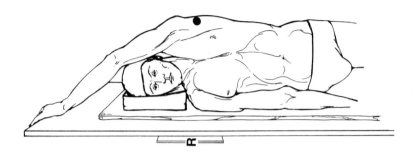

 Right lateral (swimmer's) view of
cervicothoracic spine

Equipment required   24 × 30 cm detail screens cassette.
Table bucky.
Foam pad.
Sandbags.
Lead protective waist apron.

Patient position   Lie the patient in the true lateral position in
the centre of the x-ray couch. Rest the lower arm alongside the
body and raise the upper arm above the head. Support the
head on a foam pad. Flex the hips and knees and place the legs
in a comfortable position using sandbags or pads as
necessary. Immobilize the patient using sandbags if
necessary. Place anatomical marker, collimate beam and apply
protection.

Centring point   To the axilla remote from the film.

Direction of central ray   Vertical at 90° to the film.

Special features   Expose on arrested respiration. The patient
may be examined in the erect position if able to sit or stand
but a grid is essential.

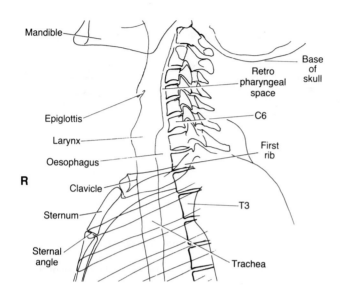

R

Notes

kVp
mAs
fss
ffd
Film/screen
Grid

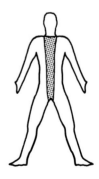

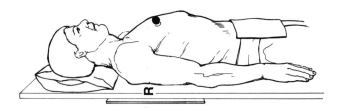

Anteroposterior view of thoracic spine

Equipment required   30 × 40 cm detail screens cassette.
Table bucky.
Small pillow.
Lead protective waist apron.

Patient position   Lie the patient supine in the centre of the
x-ray couch with hands and arms to the side of the body. Rest
the head on a small pillow. Place the upper border of the film
slightly above the shoulders. Immobilize the patient. Place
anatomical marker, collimate beam and apply protection.

Centring point   In the midline midway to the sternal angle
and the xiphoid process.

Direction of central ray   Vertical at 90° to the film.

Special features   Expose on arrested inspiration to lower the
diaphragm. The patient may also be examined in the erect
position using the vertical bucky. To clearly visualize the
whole of the thoracic spine make use of high kilovoltage
technique or the anode heel effect (anode to head) or
graduated intensifying screens (slow end to head).

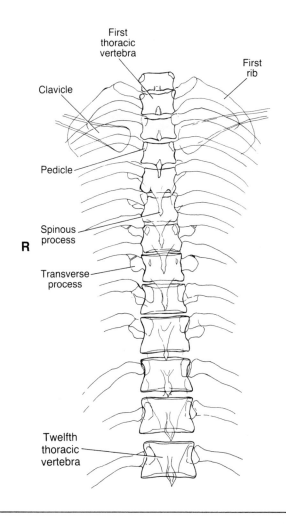

First
thoracic
vertebra

First
rib

Clavicle

Pedicle

Spinous
process

R

Transverse
process

Twelfth
thoracic
vertebra

Notes

kVp
mAs
fss
ffd
Film/screen
Grid

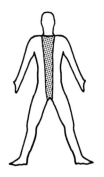

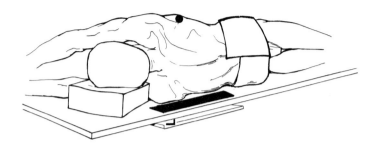

Left lateral view of thoracic spine

Equipment required   35 × 43 cm detail screens cassette.
Table bucky.
Sandbags.
Foam pads.
Lead protective waist apron.
Sheet of lead rubber.

Patient position   Lie the patient in the true lateral position in the centre of the x-ray couch with the arms raised above the head. Support the head on a foam pad or pillow. Flex the hips and knees and place the legs in a comfortable position using sandbags and pads as necessary. Ensure that the thoracic spine is parallel to the couch top and use padding if necessary. Immobilize the patient. Place anatomical marker, collimate beam and apply protection.

Centring point   5 cm anterior to the spinous process of the sixth thoracic vertebra.

Direction of central ray   Vertical at 90° to the film.

Special features   Place a sheet of lead rubber behind the patient on the couch top to improve quality. Expose during *quiet* respiration to diffuse the rib shadows, using an exposure time of about 4 seconds and a low mA setting.

Coned lateral   Position the patient as above and centre over the vertebra of interest using a small localizing cone and an 18 × 24 cm detail screens cassette.

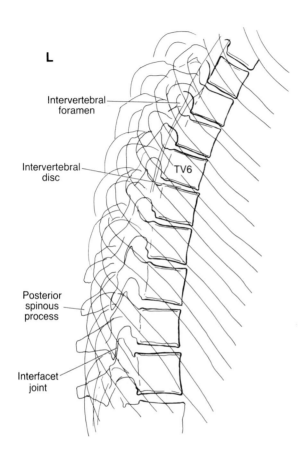

L

Intervertebral foramen

Intervertebral disc

TV6

Posterior spinous process

Interfacet joint

Notes

kVp
mAs
fss
ffd
Film/screen
Grid

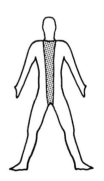

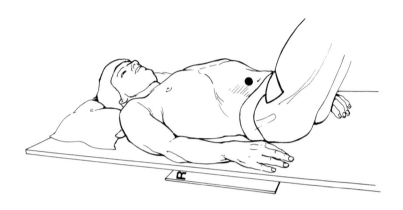

Anteroposterior view of lumbar spine

Equipment required   30 × 40 cm detail or fast screens
cassette.
Table bucky.
Pillows.
Lead protective waist apron or small
lead rubber gonad protector.

Patient position   Lie the patient supine in the centre of the
x-ray couch with hands and arms to the side of the body.
Support the shoulders on pillows and raise the knees with the
soles of the feet resting on the couch top to reduce the lumbar
curve to a minimum. Ensure that the trunk is straight and that
the pelvis is not rotated. Immobilize the patient by
supporting the raised legs on pillows if necessary. Place
anatomical marker, collimate beam and apply gonad
protection if possible.

Centring point   In the midline at the level of the lower costal
margin to the third lumbar vertebra.

Direction of central ray   Vertical at 90° to the film.

Special features   Expose on arrested expiration. The patient
may be examined in the erect position using a vertical bucky
if preferred. Use a focus–film distance of at least 120 cm if
possible to compensate for the large object–film distance.

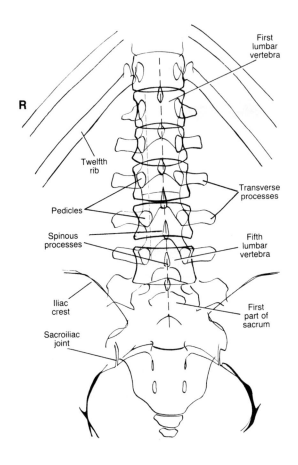

R

First
lumbar
vertebra

Twelfth
rib

Transverse
processes

Pedicles

Spinous
processes

Fifth
lumbar
vertebra

Iliac
crest

First
part of
sacrum

Sacroiliac
joint

Notes

kVp
mAs
fss
ffd
Film/screen
Grid

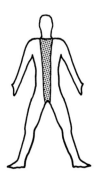

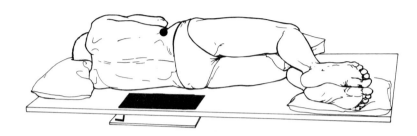

Left lateral view of lumbar spine

Equipment required   30 × 40 cm fast screens cassette.
Table bucky.
Sandbags.
Foam pads.
Lead rubber gonad protection (not shown).
Sheet of lead rubber.

Patient position   Lie the patient in the true lateral position in the centre of the x-ray couch with the arms raised to the head. Support the head with pillows. Flex the hips and knees and place the legs in a comfortable position using sandbags or padding as necessary. Immobilize the patient. Place anatomical marker, collimate beam and apply protection if possible.

Centring point   10 cm anterior to the spinous process of the third lumbar vertebra.

Direction of central ray   Vertical at 90° to the film.

Special features   Place a sheet of lead rubber behind the patient on the couch top to improve image quality. Use a focus–film distance of at least 120 cm if possible to compensate for the large object–film distance. Expose on arrested expiration. The patient may be examined in the erect position using the vertical bucky if preferred. The choice of lateral may depend on the presence of any abnormal curvature of the lumbar spine.

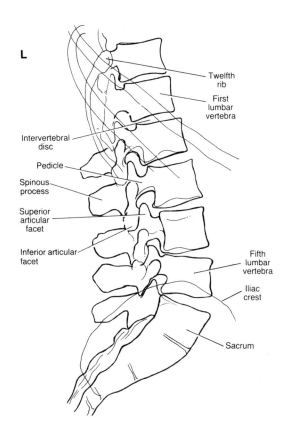

L

Twelfth rib

First lumbar vertebra

Intervertebral disc

Pedicle

Spinous process

Superior articular facet

Inferior articular facet

Fifth lumbar vertebra

Iliac crest

Sacrum

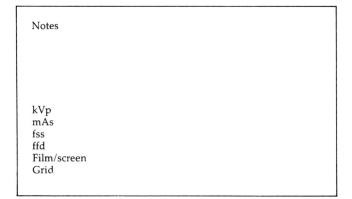

Notes

kVp
mAs
fss
ffd
Film/screen
Grid

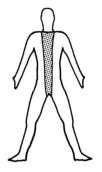

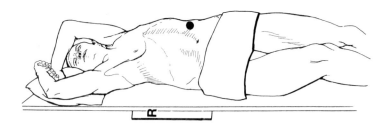

Right posterior oblique view of lumbar spine

Equipment required   30 × 40 cm detail or fast screens
cassette.
Table bucky.
Sandbags.
Foam pads.
Lead protective waist apron or small
lead rubber gonad protector.

Patient position   Lie the patient supine in the centre of the
x-ray couch with legs extended. Rotate the patient 45° to the
left and right in turn with the arm of the raised side above the
head and the other arm at the side of the body. Support the
trunk and pelvis with foam pads and place the legs in a
comfortable position. Immobilize the patient. Place
anatomical marker, collimate beam and apply protection if
possible.

Centring point   In the midclavicular line at the level of the
lower costal margin on the raised side.

Direction of central ray   Vertical at 90° to the film.

Special features   Use a focus–film distance of at least 120 cm.
Expose on arrested respiration. Examine both sides for
comparison.

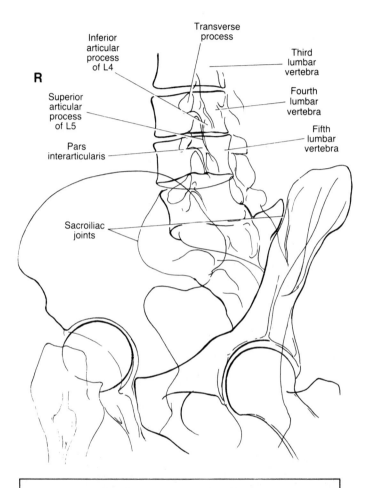

R

Inferior articular process of L4

Transverse process

Third lumbar vertebra

Superior articular process of L5

Fourth lumbar vertebra

Fifth lumbar vertebra

Pars interarticularis

Sacroiliac joints

Notes

kVp
mAs
fss
ffd
Film/screen
Grid

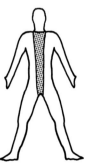

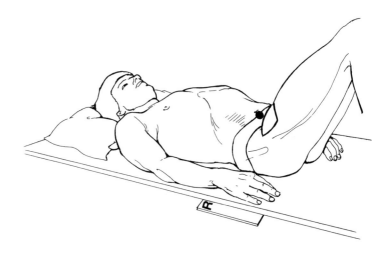

Anteroposterior view of lumbosacral articulation (L5/S1 junction)

Equipment required   24 × 30 cm detail or fast screens cassette.
Table bucky.
Pillows.
Lead protective waist apron or small lead rubber gonad protector.

Patient position   Lie the patient supine in the centre of the x-ray couch with hands and arms at the side of the body. Support the shoulders on pillows and raise the knees with the soles of the feet resting on the couch top. Ensure that the trunk is straight and that the pelvis is not rotated. Immobilize the patient by supporting the raised legs on pillows if necessary. Place anatomical marker, collimate beam and apply protection if possible.

Centring point   In the midline at the level of the anterior superior iliac spines.

Direction of central ray   Vertical with tube angled 5–15° towards the head (cephalad).

Special features   Expose on arrested respiration. The degree of tube angulation will depend on the lumbosacral angle. The smaller angle should be used for male patients and the larger angle for female patients.

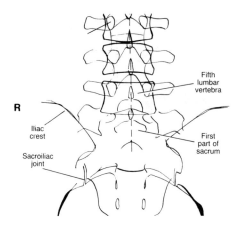

R

Fifth
lumbar
vertebra

Iliac
crest

First
part of
sacrum

Sacroiliac
joint

Notes

kVp
mAs
fss
ffd
Film/screen
Grid

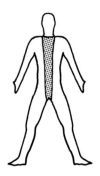

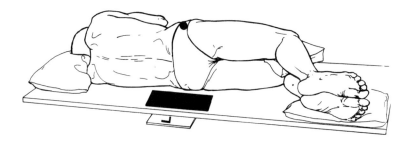

Coned left lateral view of lumbosacral articulation (L5/S1 junction)

Equipment required   18 × 24 cm fast screens cassette.
Table bucky.
Sandbags.
Foam pads.
Small localizing cone.
Lead rubber gonad protection (not shown).
Sheet of lead rubber.

Patient position   Lie the patient in the true lateral position in the centre of the x-ray couch with the arms raised. Support the head with pillows. Flex the hips and knees and place the legs in a comfortable position using sandbags or pads as necessary. Ensure that the lumbar spine is parallel to the couch top and use padding as necessary. Immobilize the patient. Place anatomical marker, collimate beam using a small localizing cone and apply protection if possible.

Centring point   7.5 cm anterior to the spinous process of the fifth lumbar vertebra.

Direction of central ray   Vertical at 90° to the film or at right angles to the spine if not parallel to the film.

Special features   Place a sheet of lead rubber behind the patient on the couch top to improve image quality. Use a focus–film distance of at least 120 cm. Expose on arrested respiration.

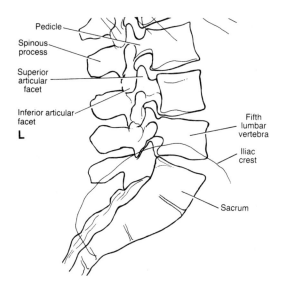

Pedicle

Spinous process

Superior articular facet

Inferior articular facet

L

Fifth lumbar vertebra

Iliac crest

Sacrum

Notes

kVp
mAs
fss
ffd
Film/screen
Grid

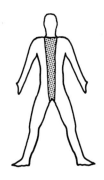

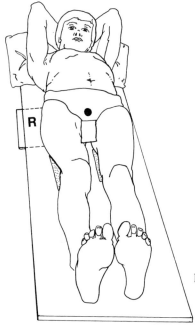

Anteroposterior view of sacrum

Equipment required   24 × 30 cm detail or
fast screens
cassette.
Table bucky.
Pillows.
Foam pads.
Lead rubber gonad
protection for male
patient.

Patient position   Lie the patient supine in the centre of the
x-ray couch with the legs extended. Support the shoulders on
pillows and flex the knees over foam pads or a pillow. Rest the
hands above the head on the chest. Ensure that the trunk is
straight and that the pelvis is level. Immobilize the patient.
Place anatomical marker, collimate beam and apply protection
if possible.

Centring point   In the midline above the symphysis pubis.

Direction of central ray   Vertical with the tube angled 15–25°
towards the head (cephalad).

Special features   Expose on arrested respiration. The degree
of tube angulation will depend on the lumbosacral angle. The
smaller angle should be used for male patients and the larger
angle for female patients.

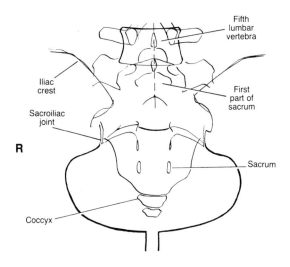

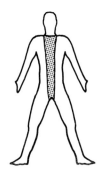

Notes

kVp
mAs
fss
ffd
Film/screen
Grid

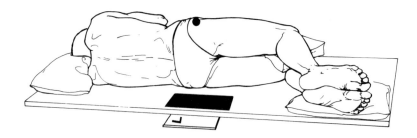

Combined left lateral view of sacrum and coccyx

Equipment required   24 × 30 cm fast screens cassette.
Table bucky.
Sandbags.
Foam pads.
Lead rubber gonad protection (not
shown).
Sheet of lead rubber.

Patient position   Lie the patient in the true lateral position in
the centre of the x-ray couch with the arms raised. Support the
head with pillows. Flex the hips and knees and place the legs
in a comfortable position using pads or sandbags as
necessary. Ensure that the lumbar spine is parallel to the
couch top using pads if necessary. Immobilize the patient.
Place anatomical marker, collimate beam and apply protection
if possible.

Centring point   7.5 cm anterior to the posterior inferior iliac
spine.

Direction of central ray   Vertical at 90° to the film or
perpendicular to the long axis of the sacrum if this is not
parallel to the film.

Special features   Use a focus–film distance of at least 120 cm
and a tube kilovoltage of at least 85 kVp. Expose on arrested
respiration.

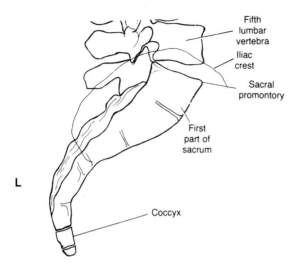

Fifth
lumbar
vertebra

Iliac
crest

Sacral
promontory

First
part of
sacrum

L

Coccyx

Notes

kVp
mAs
fss
ffd
Film/screen
Grid

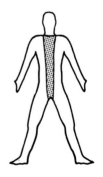

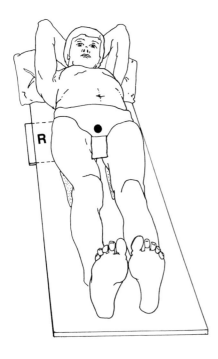

Anteroposterior view of coccyx

Equipment required

18 × 24 cm detail or fast screens cassette.
Table bucky.
Sandbags.
Foam pads.
Lead rubber gonad protection for male patient.

Patient position Lie the patient supine in the centre of the x-ray couch with the legs extended. Support the shoulders on pillows and flex the knees over a foam pad. Rest the hands above the head or on the chest. Ensure that the trunk is straight and that the pelvis is level. Immobilize the patient. Place anatomical marker, collimate beam and apply protection if possible.

Centring point In the midline 3 cm above the superior border of the symphysis pubis.

Direction of central ray Vertical with tube angled 10–15° towards the feet (caudad).

Special features Expose on arrested respiration. Use this projection only if absolutely necessary since the patient will receive a high radiation dose to the gonads, especially females. Bowel preparation prior to the examination may be an advantage.

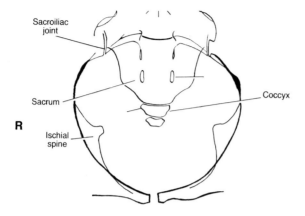

Sacroiliac
joint

Sacrum

Coccyx

R

Ischial
spine

Notes

kVp
mAs
fss
ffd
Film/screen
Grid

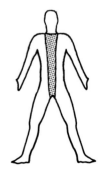

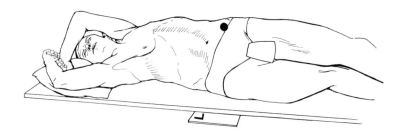

Posterior oblique view of left sacroiliac joint

Equipment required   18 × 24 cm detail screens cassette.
Table bucky.
Pillows.
Foam pads.
Lead protective waist apron or lead
rubber gonad protection for male
patient.

Patient position   Lie the patient supine in the centre of the
x-ray couch with the legs extended. Rotate the patient 15–20°
to the left and right sides in turn to raise the sacroiliac joint
under examination. Support the trunk with pillows and the
pelvis with pads. Cross the leg of the raised side over the
other leg at the ankle. Rest the hands above the head or on the
chest. Immobilize the patient. Place anatomical marker,
collimate beam and apply protection if possible.

Centring point   2.5 cm medial to the anterior superior iliac
spine on the raised side of the trunk.

Direction of central ray   Vertical at 90° to the film.

Special features   Expose on arrested respiration. Examine
both sides for comparison. A tube angulation of 15° towards
the head (cephalad) may be required to demonstrate the
inferior part of the joint. Centre 5 cm below the anterior
superior iliac spine on the raised side.

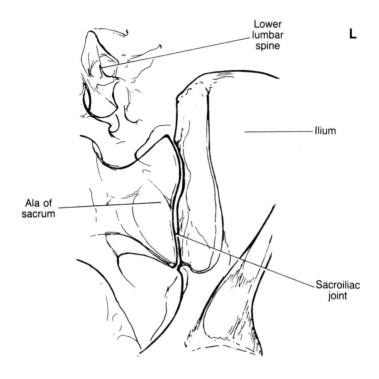

Lower lumbar spine

L

Ilium

Ala of sacrum

Sacroiliac joint

Notes

kVp
mAs
fss
ffd
Film/screen
Grid

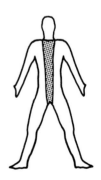

SECTION 4

SKULL

Anterior aspect

1   Median sagittal plane.
2   Interorbital or interpupillary line.

Lateral aspect

3   Radiographic baseline (orbitomeatal line)
4   Anthropological line
5   Auricular line

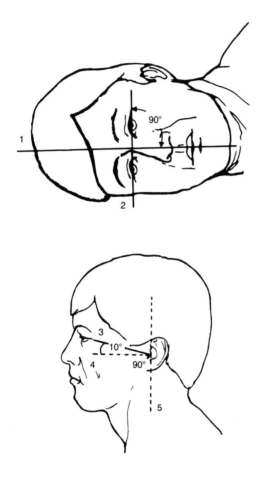

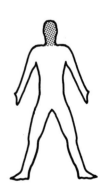

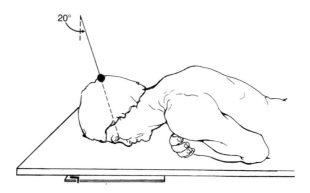

20° occipitofrontal view of cranium

Equipment required   24 × 30 cm detail screens cassette.
Table bucky.
Foam pad.
Lead protective waist apron.

Patient position   Lie the patient prone in the centre of the
x-ray couch. Raise the chest and rest on the folded arms or a
foam pad. Place the nose and forehead in the midline in
contact with the couch top. Position the head so that the
median sagittal plane and the radiographic baseline are both
at right angles to the film. Immobilize the head. Place
anatomical marker, collimate beam and apply protection.

Centring point   In the midline to the nasofrontal articulation
(nasion) through the occipital bone.

Direction of central ray   Vertical with the tube angled 20°
towards the feet (caudad).

Special features   Expose on arrested respiration. The patient
may also be examined in the erect position using a vertical
bucky, or skull unit.

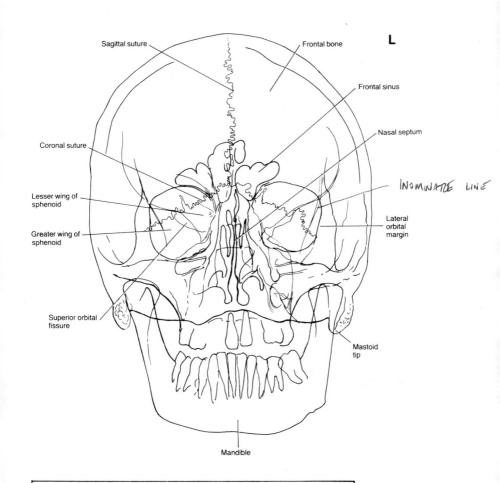

Sagittal suture

Frontal bone

L

Frontal sinus

Nasal septum

Coronal suture

INOMINATE LINE

Lesser wing of
sphenoid

Greater wing of
sphenoid

Lateral
orbital
margin

Superior orbital
fissure

Mastoid
tip

Mandible

Notes

kVp
mAs
fss
ffd
Film/screen
Grid

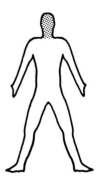

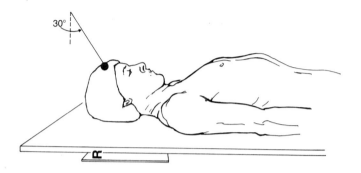

30° fronto-occipital (Towne's) view of cranium

Equipment required   24 × 30 cm detail screens cassette.
Table bucky.
Small foam pad.
Lead protective waist apron.

Patient position   Lie the patient supine in the centre of the
x-ray couch. Rest the hands and arms at the side of the body.
Place the back of the head in the midline in contact with the
couch top or on a small foam pad if necessary. Tuck the chin
well in and position the head so that the median sagittal plane
and the radiographic baseline are both at right angles to the
film. Immobilize the head. Place anatomical marker, collimate
beam and apply protection.

Centring point   In the midline towards the foramen magnum
through the frontal bone.

Direction of central ray   Vertical with tube angled 30°
towards the feet (caudad).

Special features   Expose on arrested respiration. The patient
may also be examined in the erect position using a vertical
bucky or skull unit. An additional projection using a slit
diaphragm or narrow collimation may be used to demonstrate
the pineal gland more clearly if it appears on the initial
examination.

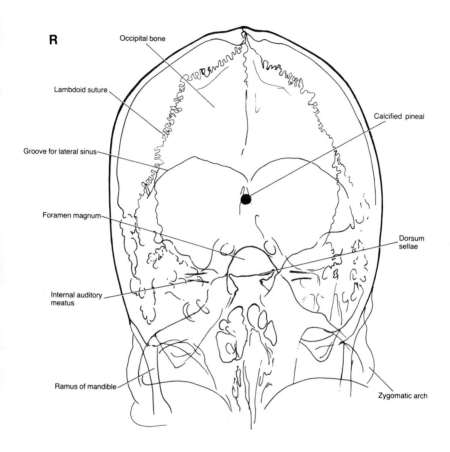

R

Occipital bone

Lambdoid suture

Groove for lateral sinus

Foramen magnum

Internal auditory meatus

Ramus of mandible

Calcified pineal

Dorsum sellae

Zygomatic arch

Notes

kVp
mAs
fss
ffd
Film/screen
Grid

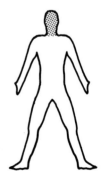

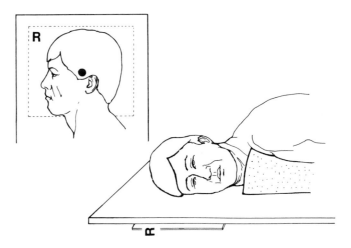

Right lateral view of cranium

Equipment required   24 × 30 cm detail screens cassette.
Table bucky.
Sandbags.
Foam pads.
Lead protective waist apron.

Patient position   Lie the patient prone in the centre of the x-ray couch. Turn the head into the lateral position with the affected side in contact with the couch top in the midline. Support the raised shoulder with sandbags and pads and rest the arms in a comfortable position. Adjust the head so that the median sagittal plane is parallel and the interorbital line is at right angles to the film. Place the cassette transversely and displaced upwards to include the vertex of the skull. Immobilize the head. Place anatomical marker, collimate beam and apply protection.

Centring point   To the temporal region midway between the glabella and the external occipital protruberance.

Direction of central ray   Vertical at 90° to the film.

Special features   Expose on arrested respiration. The patient may also be examined in the erect position. In the event of trauma it is very important to avoid turning the head in case the cervical spine is involved. A horizontal beam lateral is also essential to demonstrate free air in the cranium.

R

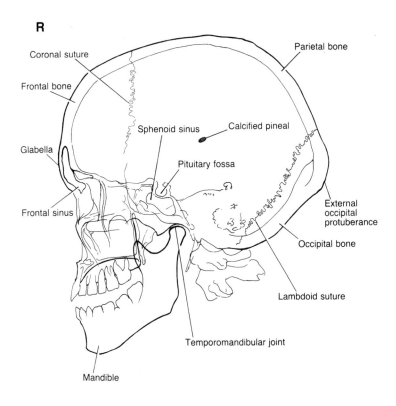

Coronal suture

Frontal bone

Glabella

Frontal sinus

Sphenoid sinus

Pituitary fossa

Calcified pineal

Parietal bone

External occipital protuberance

Occipital bone

Lambdoid suture

Temporomandibular joint

Mandible

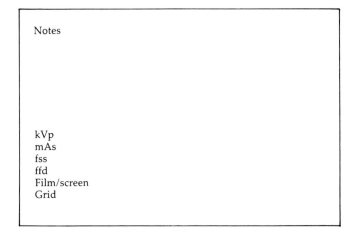

Notes

kVp
mAs
fss
ffd
Film/screen
Grid

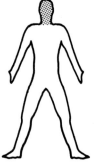

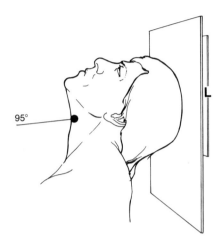

Submentovertex (SMV) view of cranium

Equipment required   24 × 30 cm detail screens cassette.
Vertical bucky.
Lead protective waist apron.

Patient position   Sit the patient facing the x-ray tube. Fully
extend the neck and rest the vertex of the skull in contact with
the vertical bucky in the midline. Adjust the head so that the
median sagittal plane is at right angles and the radiographic
baseline is parallel to the film. Ensure that the patient has a
good grip on the seat for support. Immobilize the head. Place
anatomical marker, collimate beam and apply protection.

Centring point   In the midline midway between the angles
of the mandible.

Direction of central ray   Horizontal at 95° to the film (i.e. 5°
towards the head).

Special features   Expose on arrested respiration. The patient
may also be examined in the supine position using the x-ray
couch or skull unit. A transverse slit diaphragm or narrow
collimation should be used if the internal auditory meati are
required.

L

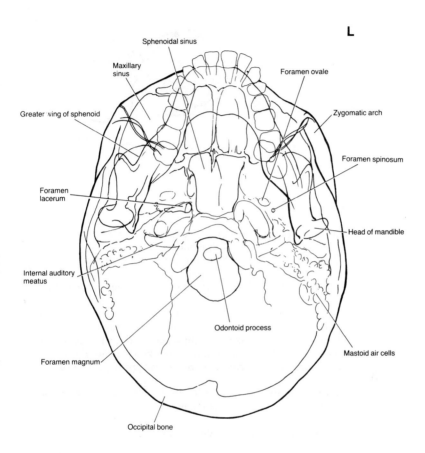

Sphenoidal sinus

Maxillary sinus

Foramen ovale

Greater wing of sphenoid

Zygomatic arch

Foramen spinosum

Foramen lacerum

Head of mandible

Internal auditory meatus

Odontoid process

Mastoid air cells

Foramen magnum

Occipital bone

Notes

kVp
mAs
fss
ffd
Film/screen
Grid

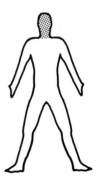

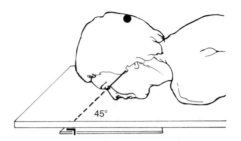

Occipitomental view of face

Equipment required   24 × 30 cm detail screens cassette.
Table bucky.
Lead protective waist apron.

Patient position   Lie the patient prone in the centre of the
x-ray couch. Raise the arms and rest the hands at the side of
the head (not shown). Place the nose and chin in contact with
the couch top in the midline. Position the head so that the
median sagittal plane is at right angles and the radiographic
baseline is at 45° to the film. Immobilize the head. Place
anatomical marker, collimate beam and apply protection.

Centring point   In the midline through the vertex of the skull
to the level of the lower orbital margins.

Direction of central ray   Vertical at 90° to the film.

Special features   Expose on arrested respiration. The patient
may also be examined in the erect position using a vertical
bucky, to demonstrate the fluid levels in the maxillary sinuses
and this is the projection of choice for a post-trauma
examination.

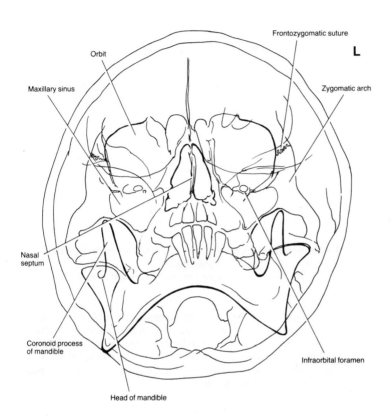

Frontozygomatic suture

L

Orbit

Maxillary sinus

Zygomatic arch

Nasal
septum

Coronoid process
of mandible

Infraorbital foramen

Head of mandible

Notes

kVp
mAs
fss
ffd
Film/screen
Grid

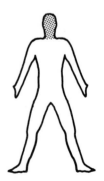

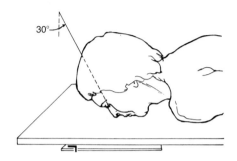

30° occipitomental view of face

Equipment required   24 × 30 cm detail screens cassette.
Table bucky.
Lead protective waist apron.

Patient position   Lie the patient prone in the centre of the
x-ray couch. Rest the hands and arms at the side of the body.
Place the nose and chin in contact with the couch top in the
midline. Position the head so that the median sagittal plane is
at right angles and the radiographic baseline is at 45° to the
film. Immobilize the head. Place anatomical marker, collimate
beam and apply protection.

Centring point   In the midline through the vertex of the skull
to the level of the lower orbital margin.

Direction of central ray   Vertical with tube angled 30°
towards the feet (caudad).

Special features   Expose on arrested respiration. The patient
may also be examined in the erect position using a vertical
bucky or skull unit.

L

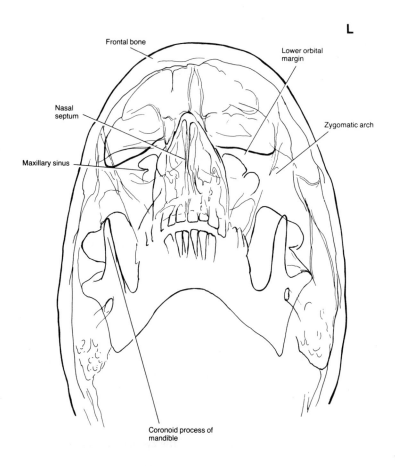

Frontal bone

Lower orbital
margin

Nasal
septum

Zygomatic arch

Maxillary sinus

Coronoid process of
mandible

Notes

kVp
mAs
fss
ffd
Film/screen
Grid

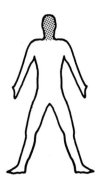

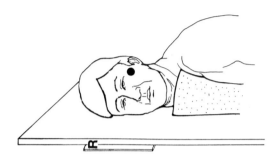

Right lateral view of face

Equipment required   18 × 24 cm detail screens cassette.
Table bucky.
Sandbags.
Foam pads.
Lead protective waist apron.

Patient position   Lie the patient prone in the centre of the
x-ray couch. Turn the head into the lateral position with the
affected side in contact with the couch top in the midline.
Support the raised shoulder with sandbags and pads and rest
the arms in a comfortable position. Adjust the head so that the
median sagittal plane is parallel and the interorbital line is at
right angles to the film. Immobilize the head. Place anatomical
marker, collimate beam and apply protection.

Centring point   To the body of the zygoma (malar bone).

Direction of central ray   Vertical at 90° to the film.

Special features   Expose on arrested respiration. The patient
may also be examined in the erect position using the vertical
bucky or skull unit.

R

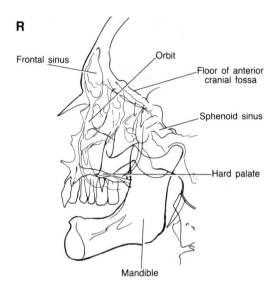

Frontal sinus

Orbit

Floor of anterior
cranial fossa

Sphenoid sinus

Hard palate

Mandible

Notes

kVp
mAs
fss
ffd
Film/screen
Grid

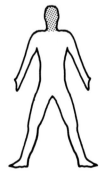

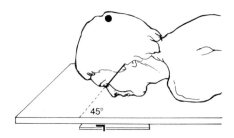

Occipitomental view of nose

Equipment required   18 × 24 cm detail screens cassette.
Table bucky.
Small localizing cone.
Lead protective waist apron.

Patient position   Lie the patient prone in the centre of the
x-ray couch. Rest the hands and arms at the side of the body.
Place the nose and chin in contact with the couch top in the
midline. Position the head so that the median sagittal plane is
at right angles and the radiographic baseline is at 45° to the
film. Immobilize the head. Place anatomical marker, collimate
beam using a small localizing cone and apply protection.

Centring point   In the midline through the vertex of the skull
to the level of the lower orbital margins.

Direction of central ray   Vertical at 90° to the film.

Special features   Expose on arrested respiration. The patient
may also be examined in the erect position using a vertical
bucky or skull unit.

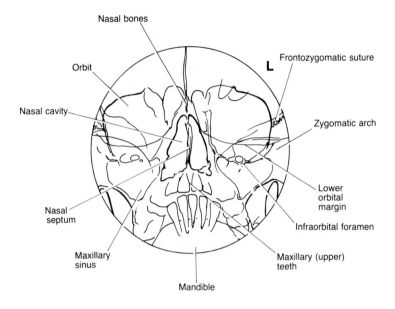

Nasal bones

Orbit

Nasal cavity

Nasal septum

Maxillary sinus

Frontozygomatic suture

L

Zygomatic arch

Lower orbital margin

Infraorbital foramen

Maxillary (upper) teeth

Mandible

Notes

kVp
mAs
fss
ffd
Film/screen
Grid

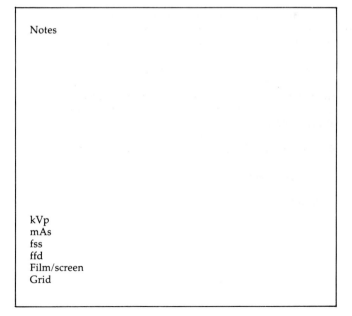

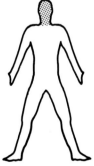

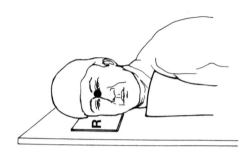

Right lateral view of nose

Equipment required   18 × 24 cm detailed screens cassette or non-screen film.
Lead rubber backing sheet for non-screen film.
Sandbags.
Foam pads.
Small localizing cone.
Lead protective waist apron.

Patient position   Lie the patient prone in the centre of the x-ray couch. Turn the head into the lateral position with the affected side in contact with the couch top in the midline. Support the raised shoulder with sandbags and pads and rest the arms in a comfortable position. Adjust the head so that the median sagittal plane is parallel and the interorbital line is at right angles to the film. Immobilize the head. Place anatomical marker, collimate beam using a small localizing cone and apply protection.

Centring point   To the nasal bones at the root of the nose.

Direction of central ray   Vertical at 90° to the film.

Special features   Use a focus–film distance of at least 120 cm to compensate for the large object–film distance. Expose on arrested respiration.

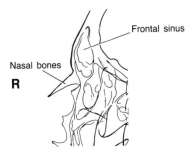

Frontal sinus

Nasal bones

R

Notes

kVp
mAs
fss
ffd
Film/screen
Grid

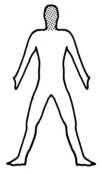

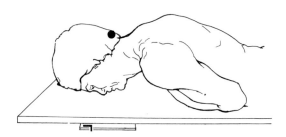

Posteroanterior view of mandible

Equipment required   24 × 30 cm detail screens cassette.
Table bucky.
Sandbags.
Foam pads.
Lead protective waist apron.

Patient position   Lie the patient prone in the centre of the
x-ray couch with the chest raised and resting on the folded
arms or a foam pad. Place nose and forehead in contact with
the couch top in the midline. Position the head so that the
median sagittal plane and the radiographic baseline are both
at right angles to the film. Immobilize the head. Place
anatomical marker, collimate beam and apply protection.

Centring point   In the midline midway between the angles
of the mandible approximately 7.5 cm below the external
occipital protruberance.

Direction of central ray   Vertical at 90° to film.

Special features   Expose on arrested respiration. The patient
may also be examined in the erect position using the vertical
bucky. In difficult cases involving trauma the use of
orthopantomography should be considered.

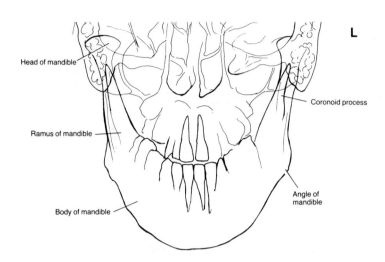

Head of mandible

Coronoid process

Ramus of mandible

Angle of
mandible

Body of mandible

L

Notes

kVp
mAs
fss
ffd
Film/screen
Grid

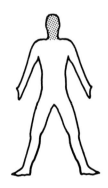

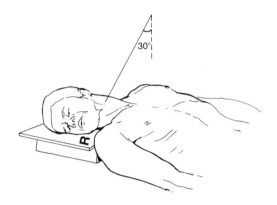

Right lateral oblique view of mandible

Equipment required   18 × 24 cm detail screens cassette.
Table bucky, stationary grid or gridded cassette.
Sandbag.
Foam pad.
Lead protective waist apron.

Patient position   Lie the patient supine on the x-ray couch with the head turned towards the side under examination. Support the opposite shoulder on a sandbag and rest the cassette on a foam pad under the mandible. Rest the hands and arms at the side of the body. Adjust the head until the median sagittal plane is parallel to the film. Immobilize the head. Place anatomical marker, collimate beam and apply protection.

Centring point   5 cm below the angle of the mandible remote from the film.

Direction of central ray   Vertical with tube angled 30° towards the head (cephalad).

Special features   Expose on arrested respiration. An angle board may be used to support the cassette if preferred. Both sides should be taken if necessary to exclude a 'contra compensation' injury.

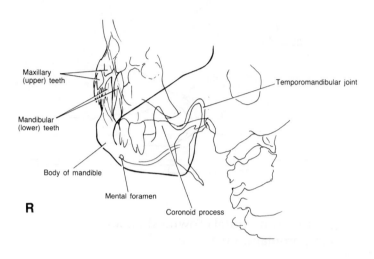

Maxillary
(upper) teeth

Temporomandibular joint

Mandibular
(lower) teeth

Body of mandible

Mental foramen

Coronoid process

R

Notes

kVp
mAs
fss
ffd
Film/screen
Grid

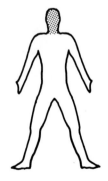

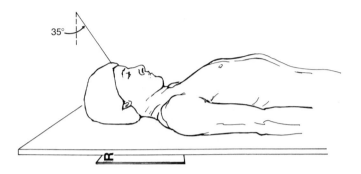

35° fronto-occipital (Towne's) view of temporomandibular joints

Equipment required   24 × 30 cm detail screens cassette.
Table bucky.
Small foam pad.
Bite block for open mouth.
Lead protective waist apron.

Patient position   Lie the patient supine in the centre of the
x-ray couch. Rest the hands and arms at the side of the body.
Place the back of the head in the midline in contact with the
couch top or on a small foam pad if necessary. Tuck the chin
well in and position the head so that the median sagittal plane
and the radiographic baseline are both at right angles to the
film. Immobilize the head. Place anatomical marker, collimate
beam and apply protection.

Centring point   In the midline through the glabella to
midway between the temporomandibular joints.

Direction of central ray   Vertical with tube angled 35°
towards the feet (caudad).

Special features   Expose on arrested respiration. It may be an
advantage to examine the patient with the mouth open and
closed to demonstrate subluxation.

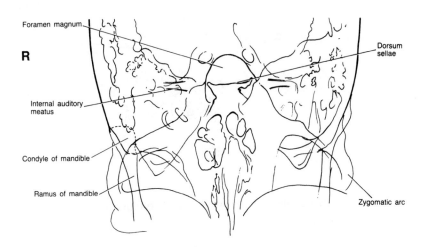

R

Foramen magnum

Dorsum sellae

Internal auditory meatus

Condyle of mandible

Ramus of mandible

Zygomatic arc

Notes

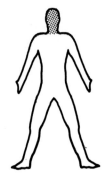

kVp
mAs
fss
ffd
Film/screen
Grid

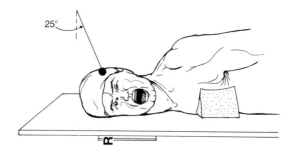

Lateral oblique view of right temporomandibular joint

Equipment required   18 × 24 cm detail screens cassette.
Table bucky.
Small localizing cone.
Sandbags.
Foam pads.
Bite block for open mouth.
Lead protective waist apron.

Patient position   Lie the patient prone in the centre of the
x-ray couch. Turn the head into the lateral position with the
side under examination in contact with the couch top in the
midline. Support the raised shoulder with sandbags and pads
and rest the arms in a comfortable position. Adjust the head
so that the median sagittal plane is parallel and the
interorbital line is at right angles to the film. Immobilize the
head. Place anatomical marker, collimate beam using small
localizing cone and apply protection.

Centring point   5 cm above the temporomandibular joint
remote from the film to pass directly through the joint nearest
the film.

Direction of central ray   Vertical at 90° to the radiographic
baseline and angled 25° towards the feet (caudad).

Special features   Expose on arrested respiration. Both sides
are usually taken for comparison with the mouth open and
closed to demonstrate subluxation. In difficult cases involving
trauma the use of tomography should be considered.

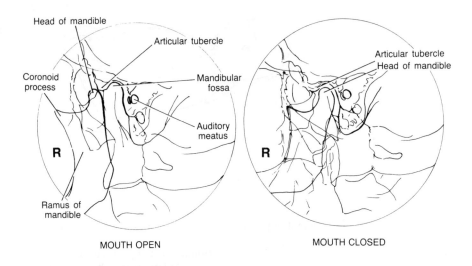

Head of mandible

Articular tubercle

Coronoid process

Mandibular fossa

Auditory meatus

R

Ramus of mandible

MOUTH OPEN

Articular tubercle
Head of mandible

R

MOUTH CLOSED

Notes   Can also use
autotomography

kVp
mAs
fss
ffd
Film/screen
Grid

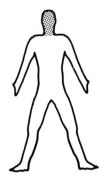

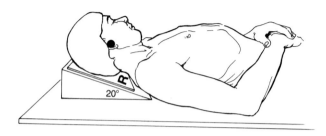

Anteroposterior oblique view of right mastoid process (tip)

Equipment required   18 × 24 cm detail screens cassette (split).
Stationary grid or gridded cassette.
Angle board or wedge-shaped foam pad.
Small lead rubber sheet.
Small localizing cone.
Lead protective waist apron.

Patient position   Lie the patient supine on the x-ray couch. Place back of the head on the film supported at 20° by an angle board or foam pad. Rest the hands and arms in a comfortable position. Tuck the chin in and rotate the head 35° away from the side under examination until the mastoid process is in profile. Immobilize the head. Place anatomical marker, collimate beam using a small localizing cone and apply protection.

Centring point   To the root of the mastoid process remote from the film through the pinna of the ear.

Direction of central ray   Vertical at 90° to the couch top.

Special features   Expose on arrested respiration. Both sides are usually taken for comparison.

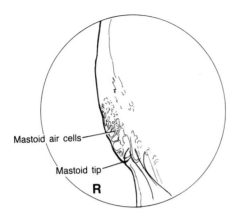

Mastoid air cells

Mastoid tip

R

Notes

kVp
mAs
fss
ffd
Film/screen
Grid

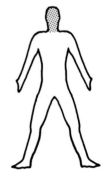

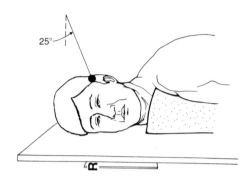

Lateral oblique view of right mastoid air cells

Equipment required   18 × 24 cm detail screens cassette.
Table bucky.
Sandbags.
Foam pads.
Small localizing cone.
Lead protective waist apron.

Patient position   Lie the patient prone in the centre of the
x-ray couch. Turn the head into the lateral position with the
side under examination in contact with the couch top in the
midline. Fold the pinna of the ear forwards and rest against
the couch top. Support the raised shoulder with sandbags and
pads and rest the arms in a comfortable position. Adjust the
head so that the medial sagittal plane is parallel and the
interorbital line is at right angles to the film. Immobilize the
head. Place anatomical marker, collimate beam using a small
localizing cone and apply protection.

Centring point   5 cm above and 2.5 cm behind the external
auditory meatus remote from the film.

Direction of central ray   Vertical with tube angled 25°
towards the feet (caudad).

Special features   Expose on arrested respiration. Both sides
are usually taken for comparison.

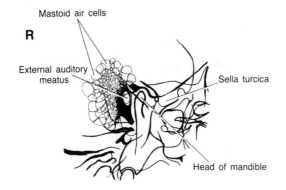

R

Mastoid air cells

External auditory
meatus

Sella turcica

Head of mandible

Notes

kVp
mAs
fss
ffd
Film/screen
Grid

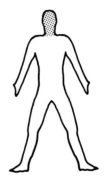

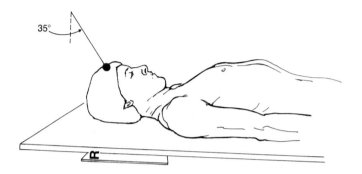

35° fronto-occipital view of sella turcica (pituitary fossa)

Equipment required   18 × 24 cm detail screens cassette.
Table bucky.
Small foam pad.
Small localizing cone.
Lead protective waist apron.

Patient position   Lie the patient supine in the centre of the
x-ray couch. Rest the hands and arms at the side of the body.
Place the back of the head in the midline in contact with the
couch top or on a small foam pad if necessary. Tuck the chin
well in and position the head so that the median sagittal plane
and the radiographic baseline are both at right angles to the
film. Immobilize the head. Place anatomical marker, collimate
beam using small localizing cone and apply protection.

Centring point   In the midline 7.5 cm above the nasion
towards the foramen magnum.

Direction of central ray   Vertical with tube angled 35°
towards the feet (caudad).

Special features   Expose on arrested respiration. An
additional projection using a slit diaphragm or narrow
collimation may be used to demonstrate the pineal gland
more clearly if it appears on the initial examination.

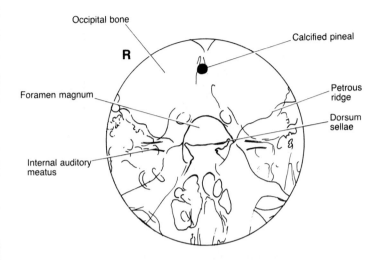

Occipital bone

Calcified pineal

R

Foramen magnum

Petrous ridge

Dorsum sellae

Internal auditory meatus

Notes

kVp
mAs
fss
ffd
Film/screen
Grid

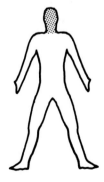

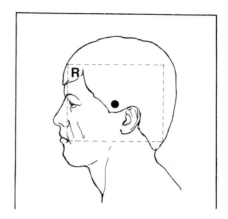

Right lateral view of sella turcica (pituitary fossa)

Equipment required   18 × 24 cm screens cassette.
Table bucky.
Sandbags.
Foam pads.
Small localizing cone.
Lead protective waist apron.

Patient position   Lie the patient prone in the centre of the x-ray couch. Turn the head into the lateral position with the side of the head in contact with the couch top in the midline. Support the raised shoulder with sandbags and pads and rest the arms in a comfortable position. Adjust the head so that the median sagittal plane is parallel and the interorbital line is at right angles to the film. Immobilize the head. Place anatomical marker, collimate beam using a small localizing cone and apply protection.

Centring point   2.5 cm in front of and above the external auditory meatus.

Direction of central ray   Vertical at 90° to the film.

Special features   Expose on arrested respiration. The opposite lateral may be taken if difficulty is experienced in obtaining a satisfactory projection. The patient may also be examined in the erect position using a vertical bucky or skull unit.

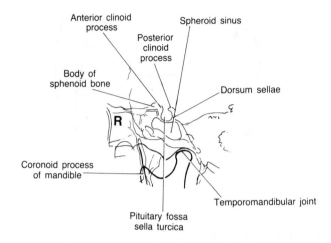

Anterior clinoid process

Spheroid sinus

Posterior clinoid process

Body of sphenoid bone

Dorsum sellae

R

Coronoid process of mandible

Temporomandibular joint

Pituitary fossa sella turcica

Notes

kVp
mAs
fss
ffd
Film/screen
Grid

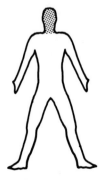

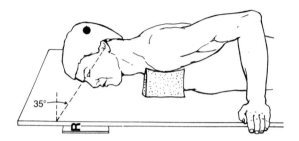

Occipitofrontal oblique view of right optic foramen

Equipment required   18 × 24 cm detail screens cassette.
Table bucky.
Sandbags.
Foam pads.
Small localizing cone.
Lead protective waist apron.

Patient position   Lie the patient prone in the centre of the x-ray couch. Place the orbit of the side under examination in the midline with the forehead, cheek, nose and chin in contact with the couch top. Adjust the head so that the median sagittal plane and the radiographic baseline are both at an angle of 35° to the vertical. Immobilize the head. Place anatomical marker, collimate beam using a small localizing cone and apply protection.

Centring point   7.5 cm above and 6 cm behind the external auditory meatus remote from the film to pass through the orbit nearest the film.

Direction of central ray   Vertical at 90° to the film.

Special features   Expose on arrested respiration. Both sides are usually taken for comparison. It is an advantage if a skull unit can be used for this examination.

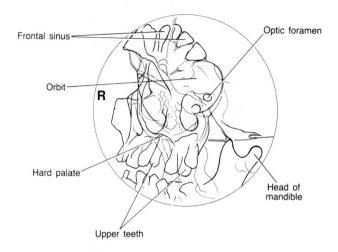

Frontal sinus

Optic foramen

Orbit

R

Hard palate

Head of
mandible

Upper teeth

Notes

kVp
mAs
fss
ffd
Film/screen
Grid

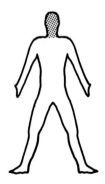

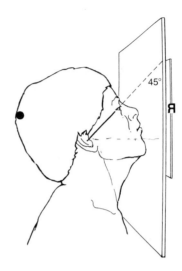

Occipitomental view of paranasal sinuses

Equipment required   18 × 24 cm detail screens cassette.
Vertical bucky.
Localizing cone.
Lead protective waist apron.

Patient position   Sit the patient facing the centre of the
vertical bucky. Place the nose and chin in contact with the
bucky top in the midline. Adjust the head so that the median
sagittal plane is at right angles and the radiographic baseline
is at 45° to the film. Immobilize the head. Place anatomical
marker, collimate beam using a localizing cone and apply
protection.

Centring point   In the midline above the external occipital
protruberance to the level of the lower orbital margin.

Direction of central ray   Horizontal at 90° to film.

Special features   Expose on arrested respiration. The patient
should be examined in the erect position to exclude fluid
levels. The sphenoid sinuses can be demonstrated through an
open mouth if required.

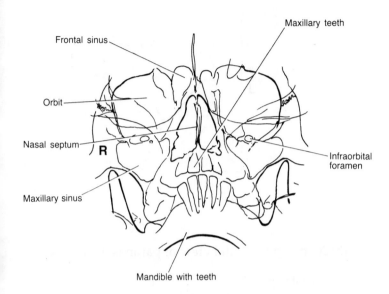

Frontal sinus

Maxillary teeth

Orbit

Nasal septum

R

Maxillary sinus

Infraorbital foramen

Mandible with teeth

Notes

kVp
mAs
fss
ffd
Film/screen
Grid

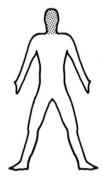

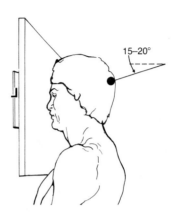

15–20° occipitofrontal view of paranasal sinuses

Equipment required   18 × 24 cm detail screens cassette.
Vertical bucky.
Localizing cone.
Lead protective waist apron.

Patient position   Sit the patient facing the centre of the
vertical bucky. Place the forehead and nose in contact with the
bucky top in the midline. Adjust the head so that both the
median sagittal plane and the radiographic baseline are at
right angles to the film. Immobilize the head. Place anatomical
marker, collimate beam using a localizing cone and apply
protection.

Centring point   2.5 cm above the external occipital
protruberance to the nasion.

Direction of central ray   Horizontal with the tube angled
15–20° towards the feet (caudad).

Special features   Expose on arrested respiration.

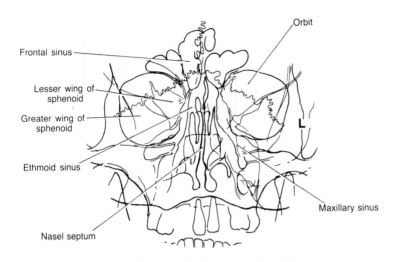

Orbit

Frontal sinus

Lesser wing of sphenoid

Greater wing of sphenoid

Ethmoid sinus

L

Nasel septum

Maxillary sinus

Notes

kVp
mAs
fss
ffd
Film/screen
Grid

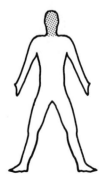

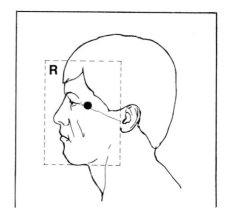

Right lateral view of paranasal sinuses

Equipment required   18 × 24 cm detail screens cassette.
Vertical bucky.
Foam pad.
Localizing cone.
Lead protective apron.

Patient position   Sit the patient facing the centre of the
vertical bucky. Turn the head in contact with the bucky top in
the midline. Place a pad between the shoulder and the bucky
top and rest the arms in a comfortable position. Adjust the
head so that the median sagittal plane is parallel and the
interorbital line is at right angles to the film. Immobilize the
head. Place anatomical marker, collimate beam using a
localizing cone and apply protection.

Centring point   2.5 cm behind the outer canthus of the eye
along the radiographic baseline.

Direction of central ray   Horizontal at 90° to the film.

Special features   Expose on arrested respiration.

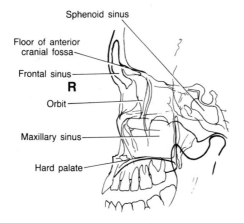

Sphenoid sinus

Floor of anterior
cranial fossa

Frontal sinus

R

Orbit

Maxillary sinus

Hard palate

Notes

kVp
mAs
fss
ffd
Film/screen
Grid

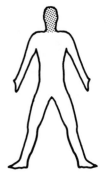

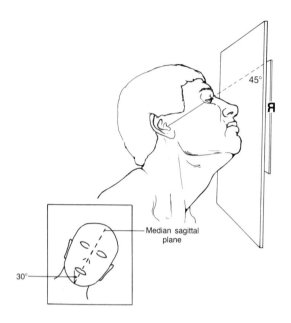

Median sagittal plane

Occipitomental view of paranasal sinuses for fluid levels

Equipment required   18 × 24 cm detail screens cassette.
Vertical bucky.
Localizing cone.
Lead protective waist apron.

Patient position   Sit the patient facing the centre of the vertical bucky. Place the nose and chin in contact with the bucky top in the midline. Adjust the head so that the median sagittal plane is at right angles and the radiographic baseline is at 45° to the film. Tilt the head to one side until the median sagittal plane is at 30° to the vertical. Immobilize the head. Place anatomical marker, collimate beam using a localizing cone and apply protection.

Centring point   In the midline midway between the levels of the two lower orbital margins.

Direction of central ray   Horizontal at 90° to the film.

Special features   Expose on arrested respiration. Ensure that the frontal and maxillary sinuses are within the limits of the coned x-ray beam.

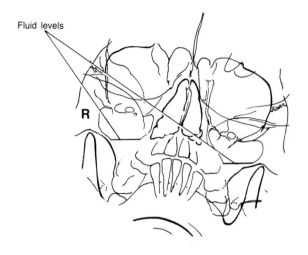

Fluid levels

R

Notes

kVp
mAs
fss
ffd
Film/screen
Grid

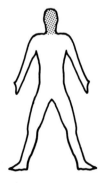

SECTION 5

THORAX AND ABDOMEN

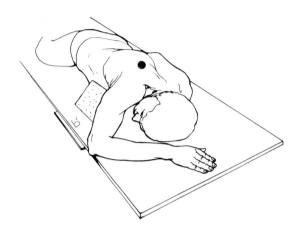

Left anterior oblique view of sternum

Equipment required   24 × 30 cm detail screens cassette.
Table bucky.
Sandbags.
Foam pads.
Lead protective waist apron.

Patient position   Lie the patient prone in the centre of the
x-ray couch. Raise the right side of the trunk to 45° and turn
the head to face the raised side. Support the raised shoulder
with foam pads. Place the arm of the raised side above the
head and place the other arm in a comfortable position at the
side of the body. Ensure that the sternum is centred to the
midline of the couch top. Immobilize the patient. Place
anatomical marker, collimate beam and apply protection.

Centring point   10 cm from the spinous processes at the level
of the fifth thoracic vertebra on the side remote from the film.

Direction of central ray   Vertical at 90° to the film.

Special features   Expose during quiet respiration using a low
mA setting and a long exposure time to diffuse the rib
shadows. The patient may also be examined in the erect
position using a vertical bucky.

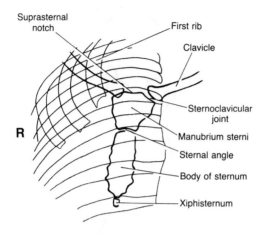

Suprasternal notch

First rib

Clavicle

Sternoclavicular joint

Manubrium sterni

Sternal angle

Body of sternum

Xiphisternum

R

Notes

kVp
mAs
fss
ffd
Film/screen
Grid

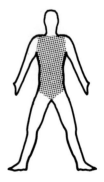

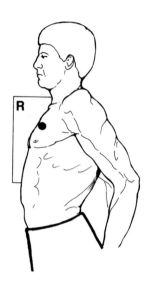

Right lateral view of sternum

Equipment required   24 × 30 cm detail screens cassette.
Vertical cassette stand.
Lead protective waist apron.

Patient position   Stand the patient erect in the true lateral
position against the vertical cassette stand. Separate the feet,
move the shoulders well back and place the hands behind the
lower back. Immobilize the patient. Place anatomical marker,
collimate beam and apply protection.

Centring point   Sternal angle.

Direction of central ray   Horizontal at 90° to the film.

Special features   Expose on arrested respiration. Use a
focus–film distance of at least 150 cm to compensate for the
large object–film distance.

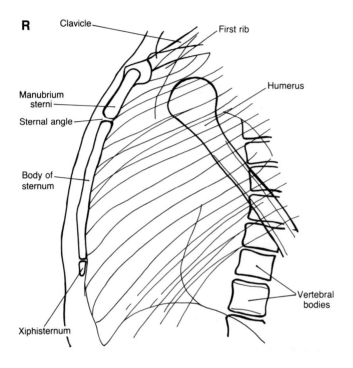

R

Clavicle

First rib

Manubrium sterni

Humerus

Sternal angle

Body of sternum

Vertebral bodies

Xiphisternum

Notes

kVp
mAs
fss
ffd
Film/screen
Grid

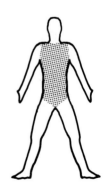

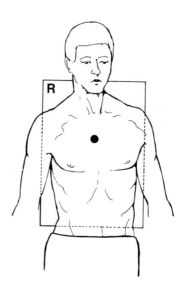

Anteroposterior view of upper ribs

Equipment required   25 × 43 cm detail screens cassette.
Vertical cassette stand.
Lead protective waist apron.

Patient position   Stand the patient erect facing the x-ray tube
with the feet apart. Rest the back in contact with the cassette.
Bring the upper arms forward and rest the backs of the hands
on hips. Ensure that the upper edge of the cassette is at least
2.5 cm above the root of the neck. Immobilize the patient.
Place anatomical marker, collimate beam and apply
protection.

Centring point   In the midline to the sternal angle.

Direction of central ray   Horizontal at 90° to the film.

Special features   Expose on arrested full inspiration. In cases
of trauma, the patient should be examined in the erect
position whenever possible to minimize the risk of lung
puncture being caused by a fractured rib. A posteroanterior
projection of the chest should also be included.

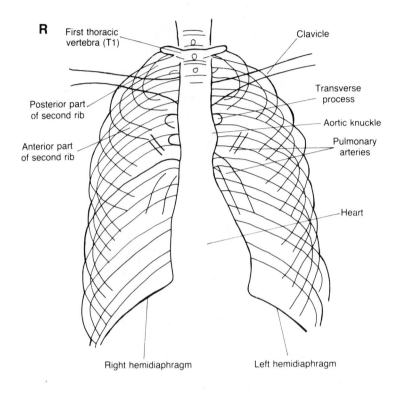

R

First thoracic vertebra (T1)

Clavicle

Transverse process

Posterior part of second rib

Aortic knuckle

Anterior part of second rib

Pulmonary arteries

Heart

Right hemidiaphragm

Left hemidiaphragm

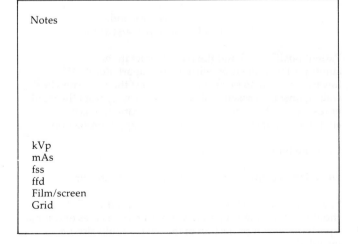

Notes

kVp
mAs
fss
ffd
Film/screen
Grid

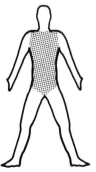

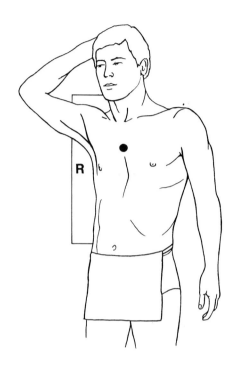

Oblique view of right upper ribs

Equipment required   30 × 40 cm detail screens cassette.
Vertical cassette stand.
Lead protective waist apron.

Patient position   Stand the patient erect in the anteroposterior position with the feet apart. Rotate 45° towards the side to be examined and rest the posterior chest wall against the cassette. Move the arms away from the trunk or rest above the head. Immobilize the patient. Place anatomical marker, collimate beam and apply protection.

Centring point   Sternal angle.

Direction of central ray   Horizontal at 90° to the film.

Special features   Expose on arrested inspiration. Both sides should be examined separately if required. In cases of trauma a posteroanterior projection of the chest should also be included.

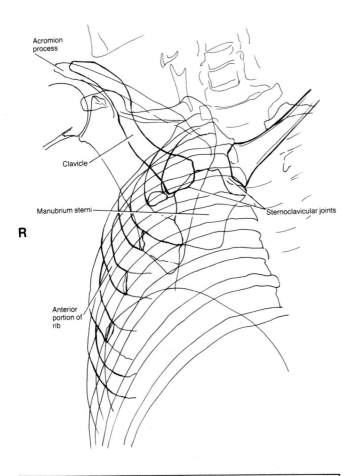

Acromion process

Clavicle

Manubrium sterni

Sternoclavicular joints

R

Anterior portion of rib

Notes

kVp
mAs
fss
ffd
Film/screen
Grid

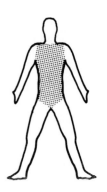

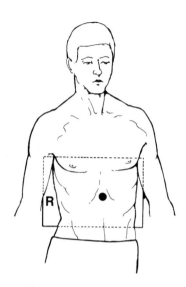

Anteroposterior view of lower ribs

Equipment required   35 × 43 cm detail screens cassette.
Vertical bucky.
Lead protective waist apron.

Patient position   Stand the patient erect in the
anteroposterior position with feet apart. Rest the back in
contact with the centre of the vertical bucky. Place the film
transversely to include both sides from the axilla to the lower
costal margin. Immobilize the patient. Place anatomical
marker, collimate beam and apply protection.

Centring point   In the midline at the level of the twelfth
thoracic vertebra towards the middle of the film.

Direction of central ray   Horizontal over the lower costal
margin and then angled about 10° upwards to the centre of the
film.

Special features   Expose on arrested expiration. The patient
may also be examined in the supine position using the table
bucky. The upward angulation of the x-ray beam is to avoid
unnecessary irradiation of the lower abdomen. In cases of
trauma a posteroanterior projection of the chest should also be
included.

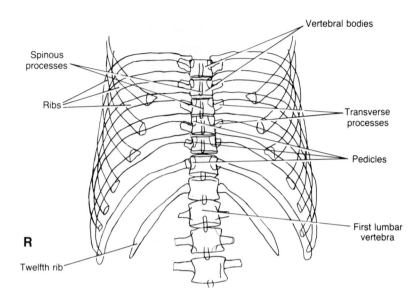

Vertebral bodies

Spinous
processes

Ribs

Transverse
processes

Pedicles

First lumbar
vertebra

R

Twelfth rib

Notes

kVp
mAs
fss
ffd
Film/screen
Grid

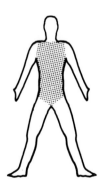

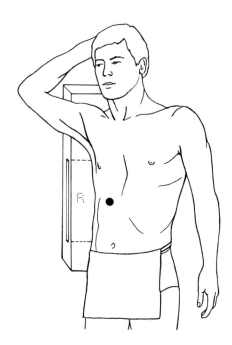

Oblique view of right lower ribs

Equipment required   30 × 40 cm detail screens cassette.
Vertical bucky.
Lead protective waist apron.

Patient position   Stand the patient erect in the anteroposterior position with feet apart. Rotate 45° towards the side to be examined and rest the posterior chest wall in contact with the centre of the vertical bucky. Raise the arm on the affected side and rest on the head. Place the film to include from the axilla to the lower costal margin. Immobilize the patient. Place anatomical marker, collimate beam and apply protection.

Centring point   In the midline at the level of the twelfth thoracic vertebra towards the middle of the film.

Direction of central ray   Horizontal over the lower costal margin and then angled about 10° upwards to the centre of the film.

Special features   Expose on arrested expiration. Both sides should be examined separately if required.

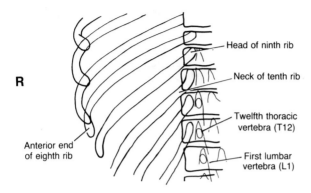

R

Head of ninth rib

Neck of tenth rib

Twelfth thoracic
vertebra (T12)

Anterior end
of eighth rib

First lumbar
vertebra (L1)

Notes

kVp
mAs
fss
ffd
Film/screen
Grid

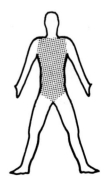

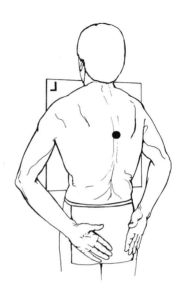

Posteroanterior view of chest

Equipment required   35 × 43 cm (male) or 35 × 35 cm
(female) detail screens cassette.
Vertical cassette stand.
Lead protective waist apron.

Patient position   Stand the patient erect facing the cassette
with feet apart. Extend neck slightly and rest on the upper
border of the cassette. Place the back of the hands on hips.
Press the shoulders and upper arms forwards against the
cassette. Ensure that the trunk is not rotated. Immobilize the
patient. Place anatomical marker, collimate beam and apply
protection.

Centring point   In the midline at the level of the sixth
thoracic vertebra, to avoid the thyroid gland and eyes.

Direction of central ray   Horizontal at 90° to the film.

Special features   Expose on arrested full inspiration. To
demonstrate a small pneumothorax a further film may be
required on arrested full *expiration* with the tube kilovoltage
increased by about 5 kVp.

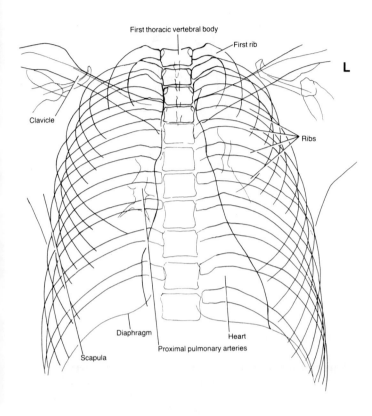

First thoracic vertebral body

First rib

L

Clavicle

Ribs

Diaphragm

Heart

Proximal pulmonary arteries

Scapula

Notes

kVp
mAs
fss
ffd
Film/screen
Grid

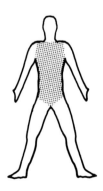

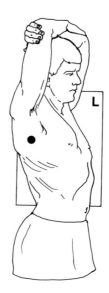

Left lateral view of chest

Equipment required   35 × 43 cm (or 30 × 40 cm) detail
screens cassette.
Vertical cassette stand.
Lead protective waist apron.

Patient position   Stand the patient erect in the true lateral
position with feet apart. Place the affected side against the
cassette. Raise the arms and fold over the head. Immobilize
the patient. Place anatomical marker, collimate beam and
apply protection.

Centring point   To the middle of the film through the axilla.

Direction of central ray   Horizontal at 90° to the film.

Special features   Expose on arrested inspiration. If no
indication of affected side is given then place the patient in
the left lateral position. A vertical bucky or gridded cassette
should be used if the patient is large.

L

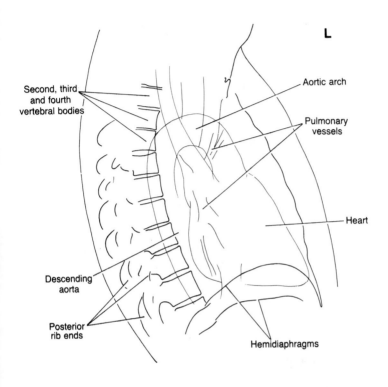

Second, third
and fourth
vertebral bodies

Aortic arch

Pulmonary
vessels

Heart

Descending
aorta

Posterior
rib ends

Hemidiaphragms

Notes

kVp
mAs
fss
ffd
Film/screen
Grid

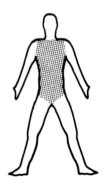

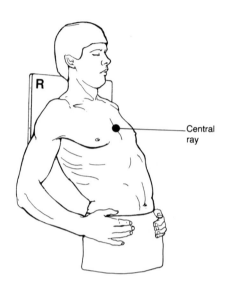

Central ray

Apical view of chest

Equipment required   24 × 30 cm detail screens cassette.
Vertical cassette stand.
Lead protective waist apron.

Patient position   Stand or sit the patient erect facing the
x-ray tube a short distance in front of the cassette. Lean back
at an angle of 30° and rest against the cassette. Place the hands
on the hips. Immobilize the patient. Place anatomical marker,
collimate beam and apply protection.

Centring point   In the midline at the level of the middle of
the body of the sternum.

Direction of central ray   Horizontal at 90° to the film.

Special features   Expose on arrested inspiration. The patient
may also be examined in the erect anteroposterior position
with the cassette displaced upwards. The tube is angled 30°
towards the head (cephalad) and centred in the midline below
the level of the clavicles.

R

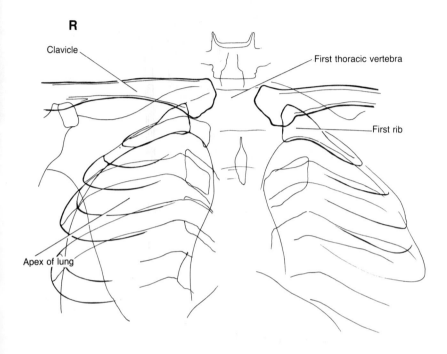

Clavicle

First thoracic vertebra

First rib

Apex of lung

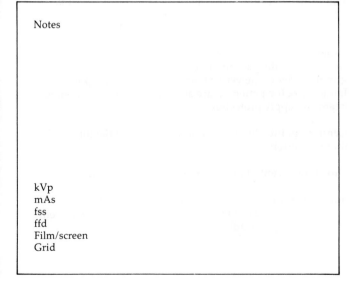

Notes

kVp
mAs
fss
ffd
Film/screen
Grid

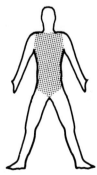

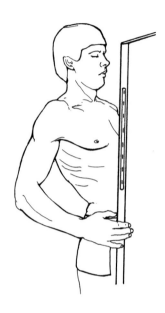

Lordotic view of chest

Equipment required   35 × 40 cm detail screens cassette.
Vertical bucky.
Lead protective waist apron.

Patient position   Stand or sit the patient erect facing the cassette. Ask the patient to lean back at an angle of 45° and grip the sides of the vertical cassette stand for support. Immobilize the patient. Place anatomical marker, collimate beam and apply protection.

Centring point   In the midline at the level of the fourth thoracic vertebra.

Direction of central ray   Horizontal at 90° to the film.

Special features   Expose on arrested inspiration. This projection may be used to demonstrate an interlobular pleural effusion or right middle lobe collapse.

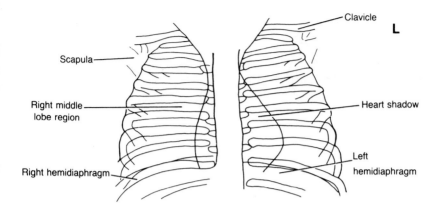

L

Clavicle

Scapula

Right middle
lobe region

Heart shadow

Right hemidiaphragm

Left
hemidiaphragm

Notes

kVp
mAs
fss
ffd
Film/screen
Grid

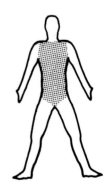

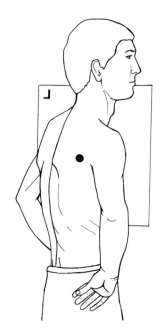

Left anterior oblique view of chest

Equipment required   35 × 40 cm detail screens cassette. Vertical cassette stand. Foam pads. Lead protective waist apron.

Patient position   Sit or stand the patient erect facing the cassette.

Left anterior oblique (illustrated)   Place the left shoulder in contact with the cassette and rotate the right side away until the thorax is at an angle of 70° to the film.

Right anterior oblique   Place the right shoulder in contact with the cassette and rotate the left side away until the thorax is at an angle of 60° to the film.

Move the arms away from the trunk. Immobilize the patient. Place anatomical marker, collimate beam and apply protection.

Centring point   Medial border of the scapula remote from the film at the level of the fifth thoracic vertebra.

Direction of central ray   Horizontal at 90° to the film.

Special features   Expose on arrested inspiration. The correct degree of trunk rotation required may need to be determined by prior fluoroscopic (screening) examination.

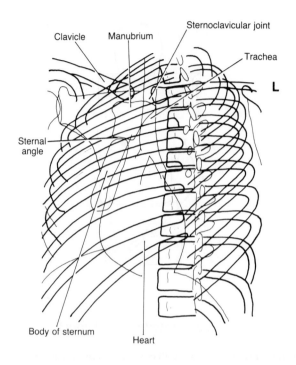

Clavicle
Manubrium
Sternoclavicular joint
Trachea
L
Sternal angle
Body of sternum
Heart

Notes

kVp
mAs
fss
ffd
Film/screen
Grid

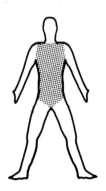

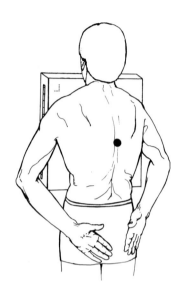

Posteroanterior penetrated view of chest

Equipment required   35 × 43 cm detail screens cassette.
Vertical bucky or stationary grid or
gridded cassette.
Lead protective waist apron.

Patient position   Stand or sit the patient erect facing the
vertical bucky. Extend the neck slightly and rest the backs of
the hands on hips. Press the shoulders and upper arms
forwards against the bucky top. Ensure that the trunk is
centred to the bucky and is not rotated. Immobilize the
patient. Place anatomical marker, collimate beam and apply
protection.

Centring point   In the midline at the level of the sixth
thoracic vertebra.

Direction of central ray   Horizontal at 90° to the film.

Special features   Use a tube kilovoltage of at least 80 kVp.
Expose on arrested inspiration.

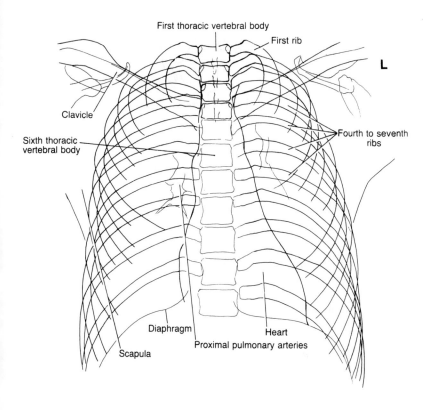

First thoracic vertebral body

First rib

L

Clavicle

Sixth thoracic
vertebral body

Fourth to seventh
ribs

Diaphragm

Heart

Scapula

Proximal pulmonary arteries

Notes

kVp
mAs
fss
ffd
Film/screen
Grid

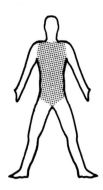

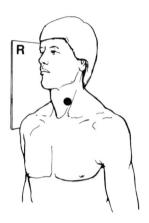

Right lateral soft tissue neck view of pharynx, larynx and upper trachea

Equipment required   24 × 30 cm detail screens cassette.
Vertical cassette stand.
Foam pads.
Lead protective waist apron.

Patient position   Stand or sit the patient erect in the true
lateral position with the shoulder resting on the cassette. Tuck
the chin in slightly to show the larynx to best advantage. Rest
the arms at the side of the body. Immobilize the head using
foam pads if necessary. Place anatomical marker, collimate
beam and apply protection.

Centring point   Cricoid cartilage.

Direction of central ray   Horizontal at 90° to the film.

Special features   Use a low tube kilovoltage of about 65 kVp
to produce the maximum contrast between the soft tissue
structures. Use a focus–film distance of at least 150 cm to
compensate for the large object–film distance. Expose whilst
the patient makes an 'E' sound or during the Valsalva
manoeuvre to distend the pharynx, larynx and upper trachea
with air.

R

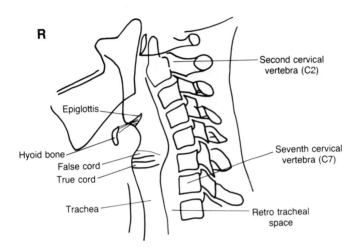

Second cervical
vertebra (C2)

Epiglottis

Hyoid bone
False cord
True cord

Seventh cervical
vertebra (C7)

Trachea

Retro tracheal
space

Notes

kVp
mAs
fss
ffd
Film/screen
Grid

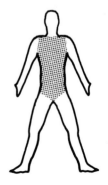

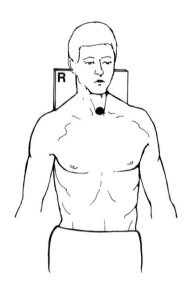

Anteroposterior view of thoracic inlet

Equipment required   24 × 30 cm detail screens cassette.
Vertical bucky.
Lead protective waist apron.

Patient position   Stand or sit the patient erect in the
anteroposterior position in the centre of the vertical bucky.
Raise the chin and place the arms by the sides of the body.
Immobilize the patient. Place anatomical marker, collimate
beam and apply protection.

Centring point   In the midline to the suprasternal notch.

Direction of central ray   Horizontal at 90° to the film.

Special features   Expose either during inspiration or during
the Valsalva manoeuvre. The patient may also be examined in
the supine position using the table bucky.

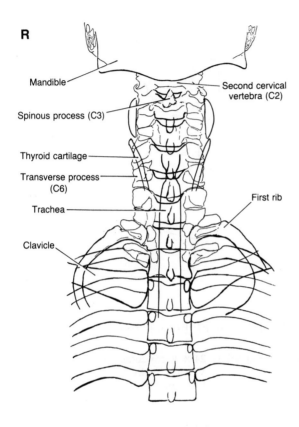

R

Mandible

Second cervical vertebra (C2)

Spinous process (C3)

Thyroid cartilage

Transverse process (C6)

First rib

Trachea

Clavicle

Notes

kVp
mAs
fss
ffd
Film/screen
Grid

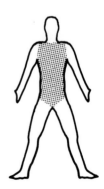

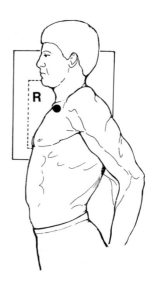

Right lateral view of thoracic inlet

Equipment required   24 × 30 cm detail screens cassette.
Vertical bucky.
Foam pads.
Lead protective waist apron.

Patient position   Stand or sit the patient in the true lateral
position in contact with the vertical bucky. Put the chin
forward and shoulders back. Place the arms and hands behind
the back. Immobilize the head using foam pads if necessary.
Place anatomical marker, collimate beam and apply
protection.

Centring point   Suprasternal notch.

Direction of central ray   Horizontal at 90° to the film.

Special features   Expose either during inspiration or during
the Valsalva manoeuvre.

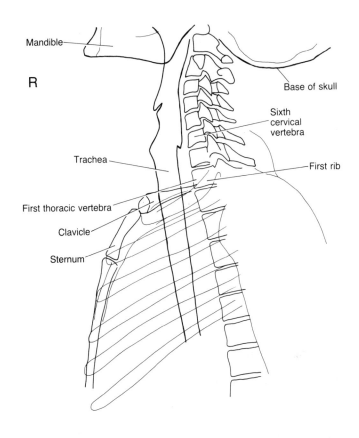

R

Mandible

Base of skull

Sixth
cervical
vertebra

Trachea

First rib

First thoracic vertebra

Clavicle

Sternum

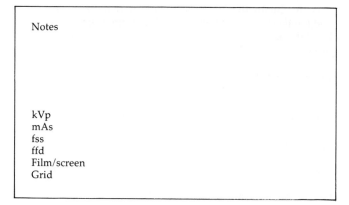

Notes

kVp
mAs
fss
ffd
Film/screen
Grid

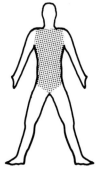

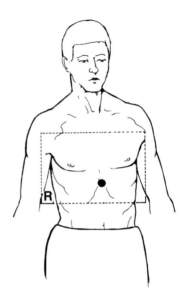

Anteroposterior view of diaphragm

Equipment required   35 × 43 cm detail screens cassette.
Vertical cassette stand.
Lead protective waist apron.

Patient position   Stand or sit the patient erect in the
anteroposterior position with the back resting against the
cassette. Ensure that the trunk is not rotated. Place the arms
and hands in the anatomical position. Immobilize the patient.
Place the anatomical marker, collimate beam and apply
protection.

Centring point   In the midline at the level of the xiphoid
sternum.

Direction of central ray   Horizontal at 90° to the film.

Special features   Use the double-exposure technique to
demonstrate the excursion of the diaphragm. Take two
exposures on one film, the first on arrested full expiration and
the second on arrested full inspiration. Each exposure should
be half that normally used for a posteroanterior chest.

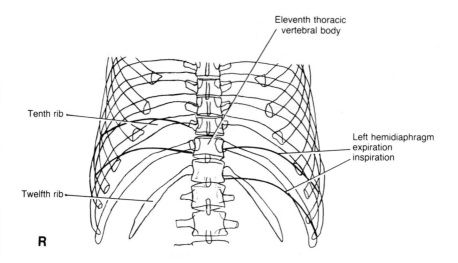

Eleventh thoracic
vertebral body

Tenth rib

Twelfth rib

Left hemidiaphragm
expiration
inspiration

R

Notes

kVp
mAs
fss
ffd
Film/screen
Grid

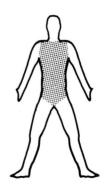

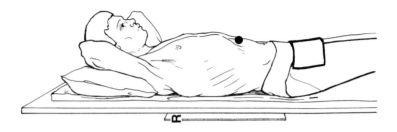

Anteroposterior view of supine abdomen

Equipment required   35 × 43 cm detail screens cassette.
Table bucky.
Pillow or foam pads.
Lead rubber gonad protection for male
patient.

Patient position   Lie the patient supine in the centre of the
x-ray couch with the hips slightly flexed and the knees resting
on a pillow or foam pad. Place the hands and arms above the
head or away from the sides of the body. Ensure that the trunk
is straight and that there is no rotation. Include the symphysis
pubis on the film. Immobilize the patient. Place anatomical
marker, collimate beam and apply protection if possible
without obscuring the lower abdomen.

Centring point   In the midline to the middle of the film at the
level of the fourth lumbar vertebra.

Direction of central ray   Vertical at 90° to the film.

Special features   Expose on arrested respiration.

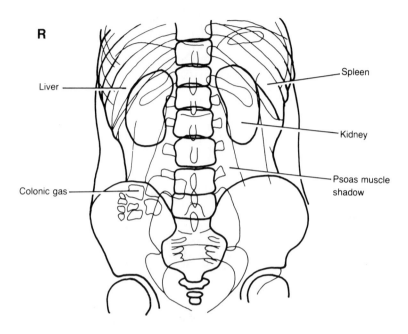

R

Liver

Spleen

Kidney

Psoas muscle
shadow

Colonic gas

Notes

kVp
mAs
fss
ffd
Film/screen
Grid

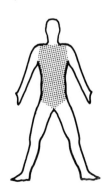

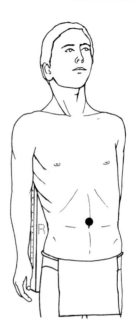

Anteroposterior view of erect abdomen

Equipment required   35 × 45 cm detail or fast screens cassette.
Vertical bucky, stationary grid or gridded cassette.
Lead rubber protection sheet.

Patient position   Stand or sit the patient erect in the anteroposterior position with the back resting against the centre of the vertical bucky. Ensure that the trunk is not rotated. Place the arms and hands in the anatomical position. Include the diaphragm on the film. Immobilize the patient. Place anatomical marker, collimate beam and apply protection.

Centring point   In the midline to the middle of the film.

Direction of central ray   Horizontal at 90° to the film.

Special features   Expose on arrested inspiration to ensure that the diaphragm is included. The patient is examined in the erect position to exclude fluid levels and free gas in the peritoneal cavity. For seriously ill patients this projection should be attempted in addition to the supine anteroposterior abdomen and anteroposterior or posteroanterior chest projections.

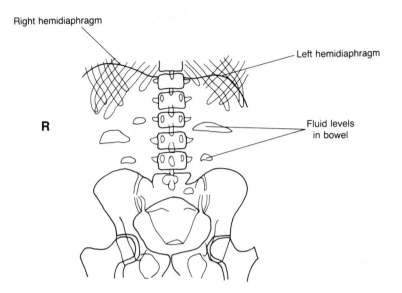

Right hemidiaphragm

Left hemidiaphragm

R

Fluid levels
in bowel

Notes

kVp
mAs
fss
ffd
Film/screen
Grid

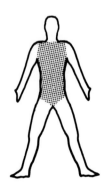

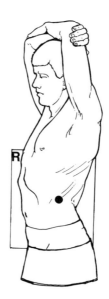

Right lateral view of erect abdomen

Equipment required   35 × 43 cm detail or fast screens
cassette.
Vertical bucky, stationary grid or
gridded cassette.
Lead rubber protection sheet.

Patient position   Stand or sit the patient erect in the true
lateral position with the affected side resting in contact with
the centre of the vertical bucky. Raise the arms and fold over
the head. Ensure that the trunk is not rotated. Include the
diaphragm on the film. Immobilize the patient. Place
anatomical marker, collimate beam and apply protection if
possible.

Centring point   In the axillary line to the middle of the film.

Direction of central ray   Horizontal at 90° to the film.

Special features   Expose on arrested inspiration. This
projection may be used to demonstrate a calcified abdominal
aorta. The patient may also be examined in the horizontal
position, turned on to one side, using the table bucky. In cases
of suspected aortic aneurysm these projections are usually
contraindicated and the patient should be examined in the
supine position using a horizontal lateral projection.

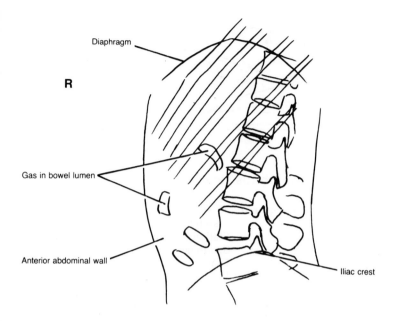

R

Diaphragm

Gas in bowel lumen

Anterior abdominal wall

Iliac crest

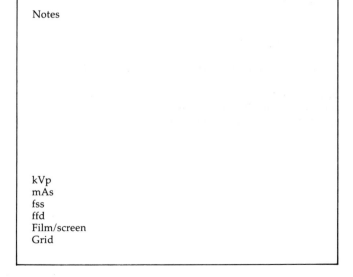

Notes

kVp
mAs
fss
ffd
Film/screen
Grid

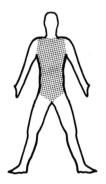

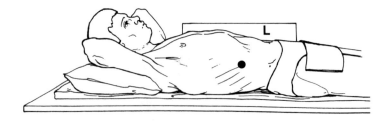

Supine decubitus view of abdomen

Equipment required   35 × 43 cm detail or fast screens cassette.
Stationary grid or gridded cassette.
Sandbags.
Foam pads.
Lead rubber protection sheet.

Patient position   Lie the patient supine in the centre of the x-ray couch with legs extended and knees slightly flexed resting on pads. Raise the arms above the head and rest in a comfortable position. Ensure that the trunk is not rotated. Vertically support the cassette and grid in contact with the affected side of the abdomen. Include the diaphragm on the film. Immobilize the patient. Place anatomical marker, collimate beam and apply protection if possible.

Centring point   In the axillary line to the centre of the film.

Direction of central ray   Horizontal at 90° to the film.

Special features   Expose on arrested inspiration. This projection is an alternative to the erect lateral abdomen for seriously ill or severely injured patients.

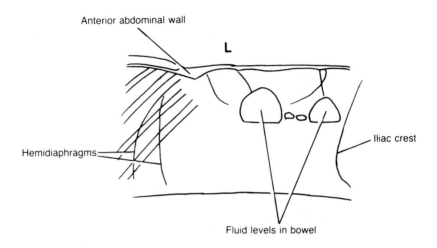

Anterior abdominal wall

L

Hemidiaphragms

Iliac crest

Fluid levels in bowel

Notes

kVp
mAs
fss
ffd
Film/screen
Grid

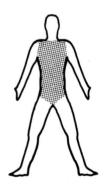

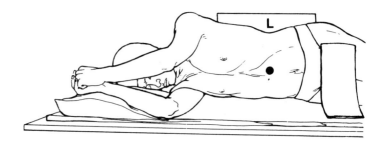

Right lateral decubitus view of abdomen

Equipment required   35 × 43 cm detail or fast screens
cassette.
Stationary grid or gridded cassette.
Sandbags.
Foam pads.
Lead rubber protection sheet.

Patient position   Lie the patient on the x-ray couch in the
true lateral position with the affected side uppermost. Flex the
hips and knees and rest the legs in a comfortable position
using foam pads if necessary. Raise the arms and rest the
hands under the head. Ensure that the trunk is not rotated.
Vertically support the cassette in contact with the anterior or
posterior aspect of the abdomen. Include the symphysis pubis
on the film. Immobilize the patient. Place anatomical marker,
collimate beam and apply protection if possible.

Centring point   In the midline to the centre of the cassette.

Direction of central ray   Horizontal at 90° to the film.

Special features   Expose on arrested respiration. This
projection may be required in cases of trauma, acute
emergencies and barium studies involving overcouch films.
For a suspected perforation the right lateral decubitus is
recommended, in order to avoid confusion between gas in the
fundus of the stomach and free gas in the peritoneal cavity.

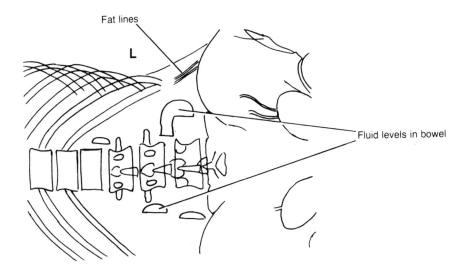

Fat lines

L

Fluid levels in bowel

Notes

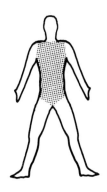

kVp
mAs
fss
ffd
Film/screen
Grid

APPENDIX:

GUIDE TO EXPOSURE FACTORS

Region	View	kVp	Non-screen film (CEA)	Detail screens (Cronex®)	Fast screens (Hi-plus)	Other screens	ffd (cm)	Grid
UPPER LIMB								
Fingers	DP	60	15	2			100	–
	Lat	60	15	2			100	–
Thumb	AP	60	20	3			100	–
	Lat	60	20	3			100	–
Thumb for foreign body	PA	60	20	3			100	–
	Mediolat	60	20	3			100	–
Hand	DP	60	25	4			100	–
	DP obl	62	25	4			100	–
Both hands	AP obl	62	25	4			100	–
Wrist	PA/ulnar dev.	60	30	5			100	–
	Lat	65	35	6			100	–
	Obl	62	30	5			100	–
	Carpal tunnel	65	35	6			100	–
Forearm	AP	55	60	10			100	–
	Lat	57	60	10			100	–
Elbow	AP	65	45	7			100	–
	Lat	65	45	7			100	–
	Axial	70	50	8			100	–
Head of radius	Obl	65	45	7			100	–
	Lat	65	45	7			100	–
Humerus	AP	60		15			100	–
	Lat	60		15			100	–
Surgical neck	AP	60			10		100	–
	IS	60			10		100	–
Upper humerus	Transthoracic	75			100		100	Yes
Shoulder	AP	62		15 (60)			100	– (Yes)
	Axial	65		15			100	–
Scapula	AP	65		15				
	Lat	75		30	20 (80)		100	– (Yes)
Acromioclavicular joints	AP	55		15			100	–
Clavicle	AP/PA	60		15			100	–
	IS	60		15			100	–
Sternoclavicular joint	PA	65		15			100	–
	Obl	75		30			100	–

*Abbreviations AP, anteroposterior; dev, deviation; DP, dorsipalmar; FO, fronto-occipital; IS, inferosuperior; Lat, lateral; Mediolat, mediolateral; obl, oblique; OF, occipitofrontal; OM, occipitomental; PA, posteroanterior; SMV, submentovertex; WB, weight bearing.

Region	View	kVp	mAs				ffd (cm)	Grid
			Non-screen film (CEA)	Detail screens (Cronex®)	Fast screens (Hi-plus)	Other screens		
LOWER LIMB								
Toes	DP	60	15	2			100	–
	Lat	65	30	5			100	–
Hallux	DP	60	25	4			100	–
	Lat obl	62	25	4			100	–
Foot	DP	60	25	4			100	–
	DP obl	62	25	4			100	–
	Lat/WB	70	40	6			100	–
Calcaneus	Axial	75	90	15			100	–
	Lat	70	45	7			100	–
Ankle	AP	65	60	10			100	–
	Lat	70	45	7			100	–
Tibia and fibula	AP	60		10			100	–
	Lat	60		10			100	–
Knee	AP	60		10			100	–
	Lat	60		10			100	–
Intracondylar notch	AP tunnel	55	60	10			100	–
Superior tibio-fibular joints	Ap obl	60	60	10			100	–
	Lat obl	60	60	10			100	–
Patella	PA	65		10			100	–
	Lat	65		10			100	–
	IS	65		10			100	–
Femur	AP	65		12			100	–
	Lat	65		12			100	–
Hip joint	AP	70		120	60		100	Yes
	Lat	75		140	70		100	Yes
Both hip joints	AP	70		120	60		100	Yes
Pelvis	AP	70		120	60		100	Yes
	Obl	75		140	60		100	Yes
Symphysis pubis	AP	70		120	60		100	Yes
VERTEBRAL COLUMN								
Cervical spine	AP (1–3)	60		100			100	Yes
	AP (3–7)	55		100			100	Yes
	Lat	70		40			150	–
	Obl	65		100			100	Yes
Atlanto-occipital articulation	Lat	65		20			100	–

Region	View	kVp	mAs				ffd (cm)	Grid
			Non-screen film (CEA)	Detail screens (Cronex®)	Fast screens (Hi-plus)	Other screens		
Cervicothoracic spine	AP	60		120			100	Yes
	Lat	75		200			100	Yes
Thoracic spine	AP	65		160			100	Yes
	Lat	70		200			100	Yes
Lumbar spine	AP	75		160	80		100	Yes
	Lat	95		160	80		100	Yes
	Obl	85		160	80		100	Yes
Lumbosacral articulation	AP	75		160	80		100	Yes
	Lat	95			160		100	Yes
Sacrum	AP	70		160	80		100	Yes
	Lat	90			150		100	Yes
Coccyx	AP	70		120	60		100	Yes
Sacroiliac joints	Obl	75		160	80		100	Yes
SKULL								
Cranium	20° OF	80		60			100	Yes
	30° FO (Towne's)	85		60			100	Yes
	Lat	70		60			100	Yes
	SMV	90		60			100	Yes
Face	OM	80		60			100	Yes
	30° OM	80		60			100	Yes
	Lat	60		60			100	Yes
Nose	OM	80		60			100	Yes
	Lat	60	20	3			100	–
Mandible	PA	75		60			100	Yes
	Lat obl	60		15			100	–
Temporomandibular joints	35° FO (Towne's)	85		60			100	Yes
	Lat obl	75		60			100	Yes
Mastoid air cells	Post obl	70		10			100	–
	Lat obl	70		60			100	Yes
Sella turcica	35° FO	85		60			100	Yes
	Lat	75		60			100	Yes
Optic foramen	Obl	80		60			100	Yes
Paranasal sinuses	OM/tilted	80		60			100	Yes
	15–20° OF	80		60			100	Yes
	Lat	60		60			100	Yes

*Abbreviations   AP, anteroposterior; dev, deviation; DP, dorsipalmar; FO, fronto-occipital; IS, inferosuperior; Lat, lateral; Mediolat, mediolateral; obl, oblique; OF, occipitofrontal; OM, occipitomental; PA, posteroanterior; SMV, submentovertex; WB, weight bearing.

Region	View	kVp	Non-screen film (CEA)	Detail screens (Cronex®)	Fast screens (Hi-plus)	Other screens	ffd (cm)	Grid
THORAX AND ABDOMEN								
Sternum	Obl	60		120			100	Yes
	Lat	65		80			150	–
Upper ribs	AP	60		20			100	–
	Obl	60		30			100	–
Lower ribs	AP	70		100				Yes
	Obl	70		160			100	Yes
Chest	PA	65		30			180	–
	Lat	75		60			180	–
	Apical	60		15			100	–
	Lordotic	70		60			100	Yes
	Obl	70		45			180	–
	Penetrated PA	80		50			100	Yes
Pharynx, etc.	Lat	50		50			150	–
Thoracic inlet	AP	70		60			100	Yes
	Lat	70		80			100	Yes
Diaphragm	AP	65		30			180	–
Abdomen	AP supine	70		180			100	Yes
	AP erect	75		180	90		100	Yes
	Lat erect	85		200	100		100	Yes
	Supine decubitus	85		200	100		100	Yes
	Lat decubitus	70		180	90		100	Yes

*Abbreviations   AP, anteroposterior; dev, deviation; DP, dorsipalmar; FO, fronto-occipital; IS, inferosuperior; Lat, lateral; Mediolat, mediolateral; obl, oblique; OF, occipitofrontal; OM, occipitomental; PA, posteroanterior; SMV, submentovertex; WB, weight bearing.